# Master the Wards

# Internal Medicine Clerkship

## ALSO FROM KAPLAN MEDICAL

*Books*

Master the Boards USMLE® Step 2 CK

Master the Boards Internal Medicine

Master the Boards USMLE® Medical Ethics

*Flashcards*

USMLE® Diagnostic Test Flashcards:
The 200 Questions You Need to Know for the Exam for Steps 2 & 3

USMLE® Examination Flashcards:
The 200 "Most Likely Diagnosis" Questions You Will See on the Exam for Steps 2 & 3

USMLE® Pharmacology and Treatment Flashcards:
The 200 Questions You're Most Likely to See on Steps 1, 2 & 3

USMLE® Physical Findings Flashcards:
The 200 Questions You're Most Likely to See on the Exam

# Master the Wards

# Internal Medicine Clerkship

## Survive Clerkship & Ace the Shelf

**Conrad Fischer, MD**

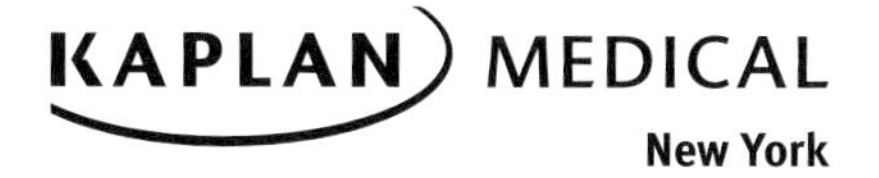


**New York**

Published by Kaplan Publishing, a division of Kaplan, Inc.
395 Hudson Street, 4th Floor
New York, NY 10014



Printed in the United States of America
10 9 8 7 6 5 4 3 2 1
ISBN-13: 978-1-60978-137-8

# Dedication

This book is dedicated to **Sudheer Chauhan, MD,** Associate Director, Residency Program, at the Jamaica Hospital Medical Center.

Dr. Chauhan is the single greatest general internist I have ever met. He is a true gentleman with a generous spirit, a heart full of renewable energy, and a knowledge of medicine second to none. Dr. Chauhan's wisdom, excellent guidance to students, and consummate dedication to the art and science of medicine are an inspiration to all who are fortunate enough to work with him.

SatChitAnanda

truth + wisdom = blissful happiness

# Acknowledgments

The author wishes to acknowledge the expert attention to detail of:

Kenneth J. Steier, DO, MPH, MHA, MGH, MBA
Dean of Clinical Medicine and Professor
Touro College of Osteopathic Medicine

The author also wishes to thank the following doctors for their kind permission to use the images that appear in this book:

Beppy Edasery, MD and Arun Kottarathara, MD
Mohammad Babury, MD and Mahendra C. Patel, MD

# Contents

## For Changes or Late-Breaking Developments

**kaptest.com/publishing**

The material in this book is up-to-date at the time of publication. However, changes may have been instituted after this book was published. If there are any important late-breaking developments—or any changes or corrections to the materials in this book—we will post that information online at *kaptest.com/publishing*.

# How to Use This Book

Patients do not start by telling you, "I have a pulmonary embolism." Instead they say, "I am short of breath."

Just like in real life, *Master the Wards* approaches diseases from the point of view of (1) how they present to the emergency department or ambulatory center, and (2) how you will assess starting with the chief complaint.

Each disease is presented by name, but each section starts with the most frequent chief complaint, then quickly tells you how to assess each patient.

Next we show you:

- Who needs immediate treatment before testing?
- What is the differential? What caused the problem?
- What tests do I need first?

You can use a standard textbook to start each disease with the etiology and underlying cause.

*Master the Wards* is not exclusively a Step 2 USMLE or COMLEX Part II book. There is no doubt it will help you in this area—and we have included tips that will raise your score while you are learning medicine. But that is not the primary objective of the book.

The primary objective, besides keeping you from having arrhythmias on rounds, is to put you in the position of ordinary day-to-day work and management on the hospital floor, in the emergency department, and at the clinic.

Thus we include some doses of medications, fluids, and oxygen. Doses are not tested on the USMLE and COMLEX exams, but they are critical on the wards: You cannot know when to add a second drug unless you know the maximum dose of the drug you are using.

Do **not** show up to rounds without having looked up the doses of the medications being used by your patient.

Do not look ignorant in front of your attending. Keep *Master the Wards* in your pocket. Read it for 10 minutes prior to seeing the patient. Know what to ask, and ace your Medicine clerkship.

Okay, let's go!

Conrad Fischer, MD

# Introduction

It is day 1 of your Medicine rotation. You show up early, but you do not know where to go. You are not sure where you will be assigned. You do not know which team you will be placed on or what your attending or residents will want.

This book is about fear. Your fear. The fear of making a mistake, of taking an incorrect action, of looking like an idiot in front of your team—or your patient.

*Master the Wards* is designed to free you from fear. It is based on my 25 years on the medical wards as a supervising physician, teacher, evaluation and letter writer, and most of all, on my own third and fourth years of medical school experience, where, mostly, I felt stupid. I have never, ever forgotten what it felt like to be uncertain on the wards about the expectations of my own residents and attending.

To your attending, certain steps seem "ridiculously obvious" (e.g., looking at the chest x-ray yourself for a pneumonia case, reading the EKG for a chest pain case, or knowing the platelet count for a bleeding person). As a new student you will think, "I am new here. If you had told me you wanted me to know the coagulation test in variceal bleeding prior to rounds, I would have checked. I did not know."

This book is designed to transform "I did not know—I am sorry" into "The EKG showed..." or "The chest x-ray showed..."

## Expectations

The first few days of every rotation are spent learning the expectations of your team in each specialty:

- Psychiatry attendings must know the social history and living situation.
- ICU attendings insist you know the blood gas and chest x-ray on rounds.
- Pediatric attendings want to know if you talked to the family.
- Internal Medicine attendings will insist you know the labs and the medications.
- Surgery attendings want the consent form and may laugh at you if you dwell on labs or social history.

In other words, each specialty wants something different from you. And you—a brand-new student on perhaps your very first clinical rotation—are expected to get it right from the first case. It is totally unfair.

Too bad. That is the way the system is. Medical training is not "fair."

The resident and attending will barely remember this is new for you. They will think, "There is always a student here. Why can't they get it right?" They will have a hard time remembering this is your first rotation in medicine—that you are new and simply do not know what is expected.

This book is about accommodating earlier; not making mistakes; and shortening the "acclimatization process" to essentially zero time.

## Learn the Medicine & Save Your Skin

*Master the Wards* combines both the advice of those on current third- and fourth-year rotations and the expectations of your residents and teaching attending. This book will tell you, disease by disease:

- "This is what you MUST know for this case."
- "This is what you will be asked."
- "This is the most common mistake for this case."
- "This is the thing a student forgets most often for this case."

It encapsulates in <10 minutes' reading BEFORE you go on rounds with your team:

- The most essential things to know on each case prior to presenting
- The questions you will be asked, how to manage demanding attendings
- How not to look like an idiot
- What are the most common mistakes a student makes—and how you can avoid them.

Each disease topic begins with how the patient presents, not the etiology and underlying cause. The causes will be described, but they are not first in line because that is not how life on the wards really is.

We include essential "Round Savers" and "Things You Will Be Asked on Rounds" to help you protect yourself. Shared by other students currently on their medicine rotation, these tips will guide you as to what mistakes they made, and how you can avoid them. Likewise, we also specify "How Not to Kill Your Patient," because you need to know!

*Master the Wards* is designed so you can be "pre-wrong." Instead of being wrong in front of others on rounds, we will tell you how you will be wrong in advance; then when it really counts, you will be right. You will have the critical piece of lab data, history, physical exam, or social history that is indispensable for each specific disease.

You only have one chance to make a first impression. *Master the Wards* is designed so you will "get it right" from the very first case.

## Get Started

First, read the General Information section at the beginning of the book. Then, move on to the disease-specific portion, which will tell you what your resident and attending will want out of you as a third-year student, both on the wards and in an ambulatory setting (should your third- or fourth-year Medicine rotation also take you to clinic).

If you follow this advice, you will get it right the first time. You will not embarrass yourself. If you do make a mistake, we tell you how to gracefully fix it and have a great rotation in Internal Medicine.

If you follow the plan outlined for you in *Master the Wards*, you won't waste your energy on fear, anxiety, useless efforts, and panic. Instead, you'll be able to use your energy to study, to connect emotionally with patients and their families, and to learn medicine.

If emotions, thoughts, and time were a "materiality" that could be weighed, measured, and monetized, *Master the Wards* is the equivalent of taking thousands of dollars of wasted money and using it to buy knowledge, wisdom, and happiness.

# General Information on How to Survive the Internal Medicine Clerkship

## Starting the Day Off Clean

- Before the start of your Internal Medicine rotation, try to get a few key things for yourself: a stethoscope, penlight, a good black ink pen, and a small notepad to jot down things. Also have a small pocket reference book on drugs and common diseases.
- Review drugs, including trade names and mechanism of action.
- For USMLE Step 1, you mainly focused on diseases. As you start your rotations and preparations to study for Step 2, you'll need to start learning the steps on how to manage and treat the patient. After all, this is our goal. Know how to treat a patient if the first-line options are not working. Ask yourself what would be the second or third option, and so forth. Look them up!
- Be on time. Make a good impression by being on time even if you know your attending and residents are running late. It may seem like they do not notice, but they do.
- Dress in clean business casual attire unless told otherwise. You want to make a good first and last impression by looking your best. Wearing a stained shirt and creased pants is unacceptable and disrespectful not only to your team but to your patients.

## Patient Encounter

- Though it may seem like you play a minimal role in the medical team, it is actually the medical students that spend the most time with the patients. How?
  - You will be the one taking a careful and detailed history and physical before a patient is admitted. Use this to your advantage.
  - Introduce yourself before diving into the chief complaint. A simple hello and identification of who you are goes a long way. Not only will this help you build a rapport with patients; it also helps to put them at ease.
- How you interview the patient determines how he or she will respond to you. Even the setup for the interview is important, e.g., sitting at the same level as the patient. There are times where this is not possible, but you should at least try to make up for it in other ways.
- Have a systematic approach on how you will go through the history and physical. The more open-ended questions you ask, the more you will be able to elicit from the patient. You want to get as much information as possible pertaining to the presenting illness, as this will direct your differential diagnosis and management.
- As you interview the patient, always anticipate what you are going to ask next and have some working differentials that you can rule in or rule out.
- Actively listen to what your patients say. *This cannot be stressed enough.* There is subtle information that you may miss if you "talk over" your patients.
- The more information you are able to gather from patients on the *why's, how's, where's,* and so forth, the easier it will

be on the medical team, as they will not have to keep bothering the patient with the same questions.

- No matter how many patients you get to see, treat each one as a person, not as a "disease." Patients are in a vulnerable state and often look up to doctors for help and advice.

## Your Workday

- Like it or not, there will be some type of "scut work" in your workday (e.g., looking up lab values). These tasks may seem mundane, but you should take the opportunity to learn the task at hand. Lab values, after all, are something you'll need to use every day.
- During grand rounds, the way to make a good impression on your attending is by knowing your patient really well. When an attending asks a difficult question on the presenting illness and you get the answer wrong, do not feel discouraged. It should make you realize that there is so much more to learn about your patient. Take the opportunity to do so.
- When writing progress notes, try to be efficient, concise, and accurate. At first it may take you a very long time to write even one progress note, but as you become familiar with the formatting, they will come with ease. Try to learn the abbreviations for common physical findings.
    - Have your intern and resident evaluate and critique your progress note. This way you know what they are looking for the next time you write a note.

- If you do not understand how the medical team is managing the patient, *ask*. Often when there is some free time, the attending or resident will explain to you why a certain drug or procedure was selected over other options.
- Besides learning on the floor, you are also trying to ease the medical team's workload. Therefore, if you can follow up on your patient's diagnostic reports and labs and have the results ready, you help make the interns and residents happy. Doing so also shows that you are paying attention to your patient. Lastly, it helps give you a sense of how the patient's illness is managed, and what the complications are.
- What to do when you finish your work early? Always try to assist your team in other areas. If there is really nothing to do, take the opportunity to go watch a procedure that interests you. You never know—you may be asked to assist.
    - Make sure to ask your resident if you can do a procedure. Usually the resident will supervise; if you are proficient at it after several times, the resident may authorize you to do the procedure by yourself.

## End of the Day

- So, you come home tired from running around, and all you want to do is just eat and sleep, right? No!
    - Always set up some time to study your patient's disease and treatment, even if it is just 30 minutes a day. This is the time to learn the trade names of the drugs you heard throughout the day, and to solidify the jumbled mess that is your knowledge about a disease into a more coherent form.
    - You will be surprised how things come together when, instead of just memorization points in the textbook, you have an actual patient before you as your teacher.

- Yes, finding enough time during the day is a struggle, but try to squeeze in time to do something fun and not medicine-related. That includes keeping in touch with friends and family. However, if it is a choice between the medicine and the fun, choose the medicine. On days when you are upset, you will find that it is usually your friends and family who remind you why you first got into medicine.

# Cardiology 1

## Chest Pain

Since fewer than 10% of patients arriving in the emergency department with chest pain actually have a myocardial infarction, it is critical to know whose chest pain is "real" and whose is less dangerous. For any patient's chief complaint, you must ask the details of the presenting symptoms. Always ask:

- When did the pain start?
- Does it get better or worse with a change in position or breathing?
- How long did it last?
- Did anything make it better or worse? (e.g., rest or exertion)
- What is the "quality" of the pain? (e.g., sharp vs. dull, squeezing vs. pinpoint)
- Does the pain radiate to other body parts?
- Were any medications used?

To evaluate for chest pain, consider:

- Is the pain cardiac?
- Does the pain **change with bodily position or respiration**?
- Is there **chest wall tenderness**?

"Yes" for any of these means there is a 95% chance that this event is **not** ischemic in nature. Also consider:

- Is the **pain on exertion**, such as walking or climbing stairs?

"Yes" to this question means extremely high likelihood of ischemia. "No" means inconclusive.

**Round Saver**

Trust no one. Verify everything yourself.

**Get the EKG** and make sure you see it yourself even if you can't understand it.

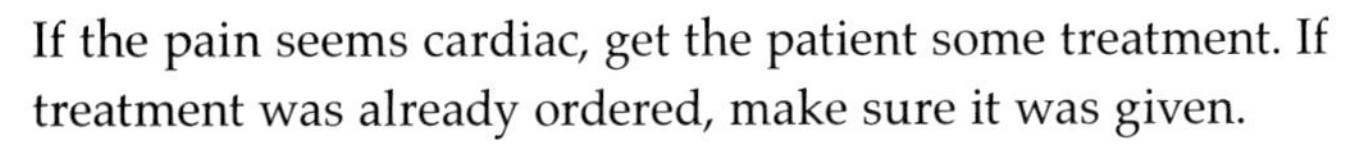

If the pain seems cardiac, get the patient some treatment. If treatment was already ordered, make sure it was given.

- Chewable aspirin, nitroglycerin, statin, beta blocker (metoprolol 25 mg orally bid) and possibly an ACE inhibitor
- No oxygen unless specifically hypoxic

If the EKG is abnormal:

**Round Saver**

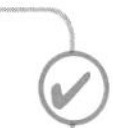

In cases of chest pain, always get the old EKG, and have the EKG reading double-checked.

**ST depression:** give low molecular weight (LMW) heparin

**ST elevation:** get cardiology immediately (angioplasty or thrombolytics)

| Non-Cardiac-Sounding Chest Pain | | | |
|---|---|---|---|
| **Quality of Pain** | **Additional Features** | **Most Likely Diagnosis** | **Test to Get** |
| Pleuritic with changes with respiration | Fever, cough, sputum, dyspnea | Pneumonia | X-ray, oximeter, ABG |
| Pleuritic | Sharp pain, dyspnea, very sudden | Pneumothorax or pulmonary embolus | Same as above<br>CT angiogram for pulmonary embolus |
| Pleuritic | Positional; relief with sitting up | Pericarditis | EKG |
| Radiates straight to back | Wide mediastinum on x-ray | Aortic dissection | CT angiogram, MRA, TEE |
| Tenderness | Hurts when chest is pressed | Costochondritis | None |
| Epigastric pain | Bad taste in mouth, "burning" quality | Reflux disease | Improves with liquid antacids |

Diabetes can cause painless "silent MI."

## Hypotension

Low blood pressure is considered dangerous below a systolic blood pressure of 90 mmHg. Patients with smaller bodies can have systolic blood pressure in the 80s but unless you know the patient, everyone with a systolic blood pressure approaching ≤90 mmHg should be considered in danger.

The most important things to do:

1. Repeat the blood pressure manually. Do not use an automatic machine.
2. Position the patient feet up and head down.
3. Call your intern or resident immediately.
4. Give fluids: bolus of 250–500 mL normal saline over 15–30 minutes

Hypotension is the No. 1 condition in which correction with fluids is more important than getting a specific diagnosis.

**Round Saver**

Treat low blood pressure first. Diagnose later.

## Hypotension Diagnosis

| Etiology | Initial Clues | Confirm With |
| --- | --- | --- |
| Dehydration | High BUN:creatinine ratio >15–20:1 | • Low urine sodium (<20 mEq/L)<br>• High urine osmolarity (>500 mOsm/L) |
| Sepsis | Fever; leukocytosis | Blood cultures |
| MI | Rales; S3; JVD on exam | • Chest x-ray<br>• Echo<br>• High BUN<br>• Troponin |
| Arrhythmia | Palpitations; syncope | EKG |
| Drug side effects | Beta or calcium blockers | Drugs in history |
| Orthostasis | BP normalizes lying flat | Tilt-table test |
| Anaphylaxis | Foods (seafood, crab, lobster); insect bite; drug reaction | • Allergic drugs in history (penicillin, sulfa)<br>• Elevated eosinophils |
| Pulmonary embolus | Sudden dyspnea; recent surgery | CT angiography |

## How NOT to Kill Your Patient

Contraindications to therapy and what to ask before you treat hypotension:

| Treatment You Want to Start | What to Ask Before You Start |
|---|---|
| Antiplatelet drugs: aspirin, clopidogrel, prasugrel, ticagrelor | Bleeding |
| Enoxaparin, heparin | Bleeding |
| Aspirin | Allergy |
| Beta blockers (e.g., metoprolol) | Low blood pressure, severe asthma, COPD |
| Nitrates | Low blood pressure |
| Statin | Liver dysfunction, myositis |
| ACE inhibitors | Previous cough from ACE, hyperkalemia |
| ARB, spironolactone, eplere-none | Hyperkalemia |
| Spironolactone | Gynecomastia |

### Round Saver

Do not expect anyone else to ask about contraindications to meds. Do this yourself.

Heme-positive brown stool **alone** is not a contraindication to using aspirin, clopidogrel, prasugrel or ticagrelor, or heparin.

## Acute Coronary Syndrome (ACS)

The first step in ACS is to determine if the pain is truly cardiac in nature. This is a bigger issue than you might think. Troponin and CK-MB levels do not rise until 3–4 hours after the onset of pain, and the first test is frequently normal even when there is an ischemic event occurring.

> **Round Saver**
> With ACS, history is more important than EKG or enzymes.

This means ACS is really a combination of the history of chest pain and the EKG results. If the history of chest pain is strongly consistent with ischemia, it is more important than the EKG alone. In other words, if the patient has a clear history of the chest sounding like it is ischemic, treat for ACS even if the EKG is normal.

> **Round Saver**
> Take the history yourself. Do not get burned by presenting something inaccurate to the attending.

**ACS = history + EKG**

### History

The pain **is ischemic** if it is described as:

- On exertion
- Substernal in location
- Lasting 15–30 minutes per episode
- Not changing with position, respiration, or chest wall palpation
- “Dull,” “squeezing,” or “pressure”

The pain **is *not* ischemic** if it is described as:

- Left or right sided
- Worsens OR improves with position or breathing
- Sharp like a knife
- Stabbing or point-like
- A few seconds in duration
- Continuous for hours and hours or 1–2 days

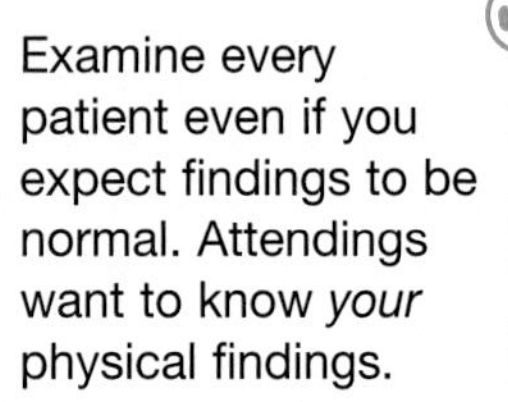

**Round Saver**

Examine every patient even if you expect findings to be normal. Attendings want to know *your* physical findings.

## Risk Factors

The worst and most dangerous risk factor is diabetes mellitus. The most commonly found risk factor is hypertension. Family history is only significant if it's premature disease in the relative (<55 in male relative, <65 in female relative).

**Things You Will Be Asked on Rounds**

- Diabetes
- Hypertension
- Hyperlipidemia
- Tobacco use
- Premature disease in first-degree family members (parents, siblings)

Risk factors matter in equivocal cases. If the patient is older with substernal, squeezing pain on exertion relieved by rest, risk factors do not matter. Get the EKG and start treatment.

## Physical Findings

Normal examination does not exclude anything with ACS. You can find an S3 or S4 gallop or rales but the absence of these findings excludes nothing.

## Diagnostic Testing

EKG is critical. If the patient was admitted for chest pain, always get a repeat EKG whether it was originally normal or abnormal. This is critical to confirm treatment. Always look at the EKG yourself and ask your findings to be confirmed. Do not believe the automatic "machine reading" at the top of the EKG.

**Round Saver**

Do not be afraid to ask the attending to confirm a positive finding. It makes you look interested, not ignorant.

**Round Saver**

Residents may not be any better than you at physical examination.

**Round Saver**

Confirm/double-check all EKG findings.

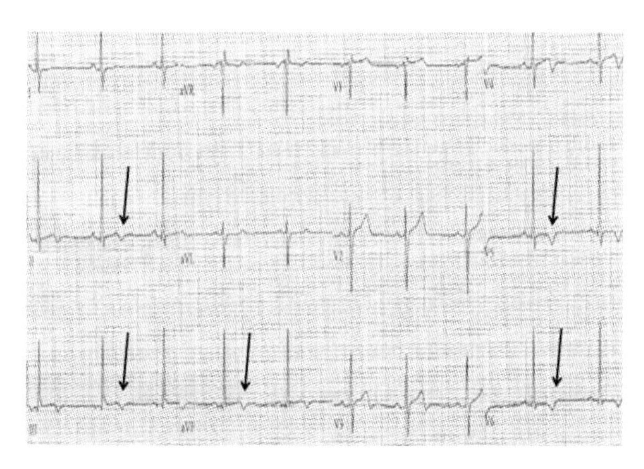

**T-wave inversions are present in the inferior leads II, III, and aVf, as well as V4–V6.**

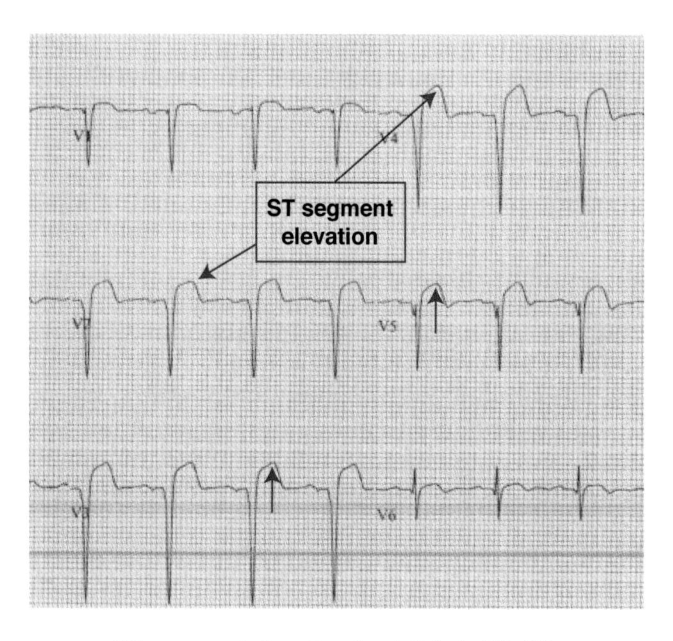


ST segment elevation is visible in V2–V5.

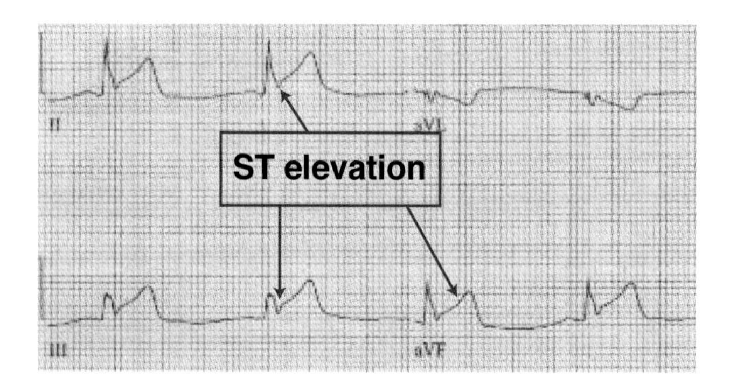


ST segment elevation is present in leads II, III, and aVF.

| Test | Details | Significance |
|---|---|---|
| Troponin | • Begins to rise at 3–4 hours<br>• Maximum sensitivity at 12–18 hours<br>• Stays positive 1–2 weeks after event | • Negative first test excludes nothing<br>• Positive test suggests MI<br>• False positive with CHF and renal failure<br>• Cannot detect reinfarction in last week |
| CK-MB | • Begins to rise at 3–4 hours<br>• Maximum sensitivity at 12–18 hours<br>• CK-MB lasts 1–2 days | • Negative first test excludes nothing<br>• Positive test suggests MI<br>• Best test for detecting reinfarction |
| Myoglobin | • Rises at 1–4 hours | • Lacks specificity<br>• Negative test at 4 hours excludes MI<br>• Positive test is useless |
| Catheterization | • Clear history and abnormal EKG needs evaluation for angiography | • Continued pain with maximal medical therapy needs angiography |
| BNP | • Use when etiology of dyspnea not clear | • Normal BNP excludes CHF<br>• Abnormal test is nonspecific |
| Stress test | • Use when history and EKG are not clear | • Reversible ischemia is the main thing you are looking for<br>• Catheterize abnormals |
| Echocardiogram | • Looks at wall and valve motion<br>• Ejection fraction | • Normal wall motion excludes MI<br>• High troponin with normal wall motion is a false-positive troponin |
| Telemetry | • Continuous EKG monitor | • All ACS patients need telemetry |

BNP = brain natriuretic peptide

Stress or "exercise tolerance" testing is most useful when it is uncertain whether the patient is having an acute ischemic event. If the history is clearly not consistent with ischemia, discharge the patient. If the patient has exertional, substernal, pressure-like sore pain, and the EKG is abnormal, stress test is not useful. This patient needs treatment and angiography.

> **Round Saver**
>
> No stress test should be done when a patient is in pain.

> **Round Saver** 
>
> Check the ambulance (EMS) sheet for the patient's history.

### Angiography (Cardiac Catheterization)

With ACS, you will hear the terms "angiography" and "cath" used interchangeably. This is the answer in the following circumstances, in order of urgency:

- ST-elevation MI: stop everything and call cardiology **immediately**
- ST depression with persistent chest pain despite aspirin, clopidogrel, heparin, metoprolol, and nitrates
- ST depression with recurrent chest pain
- Recurrent episodes of ischemic-type chest pain with normal EKG
- Reversible ischemia on stress test

> **Round Saver** 
>
> No one ever got into trouble by double-checking things too much.

## Treatment

All patients with ACS should receive:

- Aspirin 2+ tablets, each 81 mg
- Metoprolol 25 mg bid
- Nitroglycerin
- ACE inhibitor
- Statin
- Morphine during the pain

## Non-ST-Elevation MI (NSTEMI)

For anyone with a possible acute MI, a second antiplatelet drug such as clopidogrel or prasugrel should be used with aspirin. In the case of an abnormal EKG with ST-segment depression or T-wave inversion and the possibility of NSTEMI, you should add:

- Clopidogrel, prasugrel, or ticagrelor
- LMW heparin such as enoxaparin 1mg/kg bid subcutaneously
- Evaluate for angiography.
- Place on telemetry or in the ICU.

Do not wait for the results of troponin or CK-MB to start these therapies. Remember that the history and the EKG are the basis of a diagnosis of ACS.

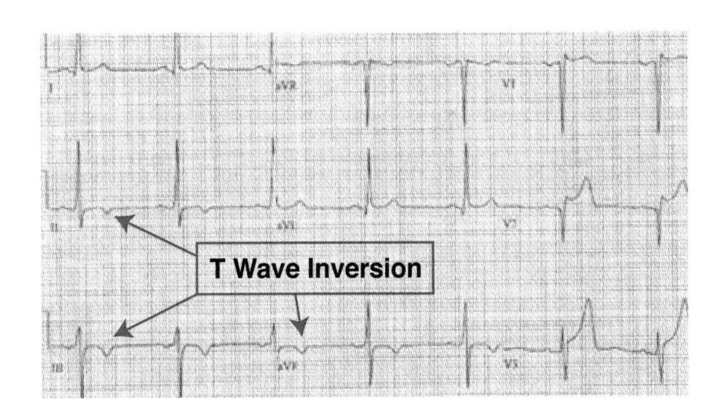


**T wave inversion is present in inferior wall leads II, III, and aVF.**

## ST-Elevation MI (STEMI)

- Add clopidogrel, prasugrel, or ticagrelor
- Do not use heparin

- Thrombolytics or angioplasty for percutaneous coronary intervention (PCI)
    - Cardiology will use a glycoprotein IIb/IIIa inhibitor such as eptifibatide or abciximab if there is PCI and a stent

**Takotsubo cardiomyopathy** is a sudden ventricular dysfunction from overwhelming emotions. It can simulate an MI with anterior wall ST-segment elevation. This is because there is no way to know it is Takotsubo cardiomyopathy until after a catheterization is done. The same is true of Prinzmetal's angina.

There are a few conditions unrelated to acute MI that cause ST elevation.

- Early repolarization (benign EKG finding simulating MI)
- Hyperkalemia
- Pericarditis
- Cardiomyopathy
- Prinzmetal's variant angina (vasospasm)

Calcium channel blockers (CCBs) have not been proven to lower mortality in the following syndromes, but they are beneficial when they are used.

- Chest pain associated with cocaine use
- Intolerance of beta blockers, such as severe asthma
- Variant or Prinzmetal's angina

## Complications

In the first 2–3 days after an MI, the most common serious complication is an arrhythmia. Anatomic defects such as wall and valve rupture usually take several days for the muscle to die and weaken. All complications of MI can result in hypotension.

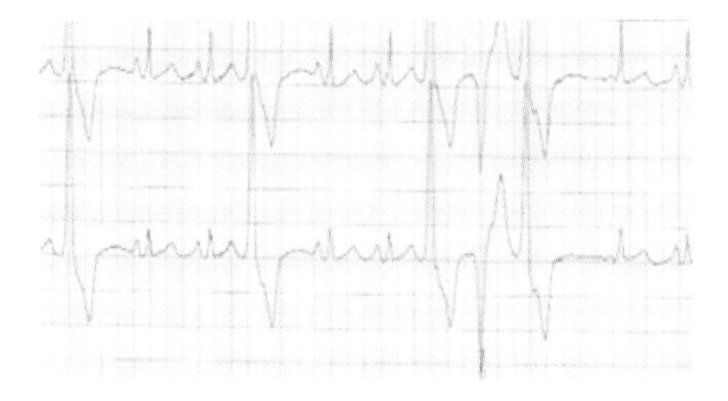

**As scary as they look, premature ventricular contractions (PVCs) are not dangerous; do not treat.**

| Diagnosis | Key Feature | Treatment |
|---|---|---|
| Third-degree AV block | Bradycardia, canon A waves | Atropine first if symptomatic, pacemaker later in all |
| Sinus bradycardia | No canon A waves | Atropine if symptomatic, pacemaker only if symptoms persist |
| Tamponade/ wall rupture | Sudden loss of pulse | Needle thoracentesis<br>Surgery |
| RV infarction | IWMI in history, clear lungs, tachycardia | Fluids |
| Valve rupture | New murmur, rales/ congestion | Surgery, some need balloon pump |
| Septal rupture | New murmur, increase in oxygen saturation on entering the right ventricle | Surgery, some need balloon pump |
| Ventricular fibrillation | Loss of pulse, need EKG to answer question | Unsynchronized cardioversion |

IWMI = inferior wall MI

# Ambulatory Coronary Artery Disease (CAD)/ Angina

In presentation, there is nothing significantly different from the inpatient section except for the acuity of the symptoms. In clinic, patients do not have ACS.

## Diagnostic Testing

- **EKG:** First for everyone. Repeat an EKG every time there is a difference in symptoms.
- **Echo**: Assesses damage to heart and valves previously. Every patient should get one.
- **Stress test**: exercise tolerance test: 220 – age = maximum heart rate

Go to 80–85% of maximum heart rate and assess for ST depression on EKG.

**Can't read the EKG? (LBBB, LVH, pacemaker, digoxin)**

- Nuclear stress
- Stress echo

These tests are equal in sensitivity and specificity. For LBBB, a chemical stress test with dipyridamole thallium or dobutamine echo is greatly preferred.

**Can't exercise?**

- Dipyridamole or adenosine thallium
- Dobutamine echo

These tests are equal in sensitivity and specificity

## Angiography

**Positive stress test = coronary angiography**

Those with a "reversible" defect need angiography. A reversible defect is a defect in perfusion with exercise, not visible at rest.

The main purpose of angiography is to determine who should undergo bypass surgery. Only stenosis >70% in a vessel is significant.

- **1- or 2-vessel disease:** medical management and possible angioplasty (PCI)
    - Angioplasty may decrease symptoms compared with medications, but there is no clear mortality benefit with the use of angioplasty in chronic stable angina.
- **3-vessel disease with LV dysfunction or left main coronary disease:** bypass surgery

## Treatment

The most important thing to know is which drugs lower mortality in CAD. These are:

- Aspirin +/– clopidogrel, prasugrel, or ticagrelor
- Beta blockers: metoprolol, nebivolol
- Statins to goal LDL at least <100 mg/dL
- ACE inhibitor if ejection fraction is <40%

Aspirin alone is sufficient in chronic stable angina. For persistent pain, use long-acting nitroglycerin. Ranolazine is a sodium-channel blocker used in refractory angina.

Ambulatory management of CAD differs from acute coronary syndromes in several ways.

- Enzymes are not useful
- No troponins or CK-MB

- Angiography is used to determine the need for bypass surgery
- Heparin and glycoprotein IIb/IIIa inhibitors are not used

For lipid management, statins are best.

**Shelf or in-service exam answer:** CAD + LDL >100 = statin

**Practical or Ward answer:** everyone with coronary disease gets a statin

The most common adverse effects of statins are (1) increased liver function tests (AST/ALT) in 2–3% of patients (stop the statin at LFT **3–5x** upper limit of normal) and (2) myositis in <1% of patients.

CAD equivalents (other circumstances with goal LDL <100 mg/dL):

- Peripheral arterial disease
- Diabetes
- Aortic disease
- Carotid disease

# CONGESTIVE HEART FAILURE (CHF)

## Acute Pulmonary Edema

Pulmonary edema does not happen by itself, even in those with CHF. Something causes it. You must investigate what that is. The most common **precipitants** of acute pulmonary edema:

1. Ischemia
2. Arrhythmia of any kind
3. Non-adherence with medications
4. Infection
5. Salty food diet
6. Iatrogenic fluid overload
7. Hypertensive crisis

**Round Saver**

Make sure the team has not overloaded the CHF patient with IV fluids!

Look for a patient who has been admitted to the emergency department or ICU with a sudden onset of dyspnea—worse when lying flat and better when sitting up. Ischemia or arrhythmia causing acute pulmonary edema can occur in any part of the hospital, however.

Physical exam will show:

- Rales
- S3 gallop, JVD
- Peripheral edema
- Tachycardia
- Sweating and nausea are common

If this presentation is present, stop what you are doing and do the following:

1. Make sure oxygen is given
2. Elevate the head of the bed
3. Call your resident
4. Attach oximeter
5. Make sure an ABG is done
6. Connect to telemetry (continuous cardiac monitor)

## Diagnostic Testing

EKG will exclude both ischemia and arrhythmia as the cause of pulmonary edema. Chest x-ray will show congestion/vascular fluid overload, effusions, and cardiomegaly.

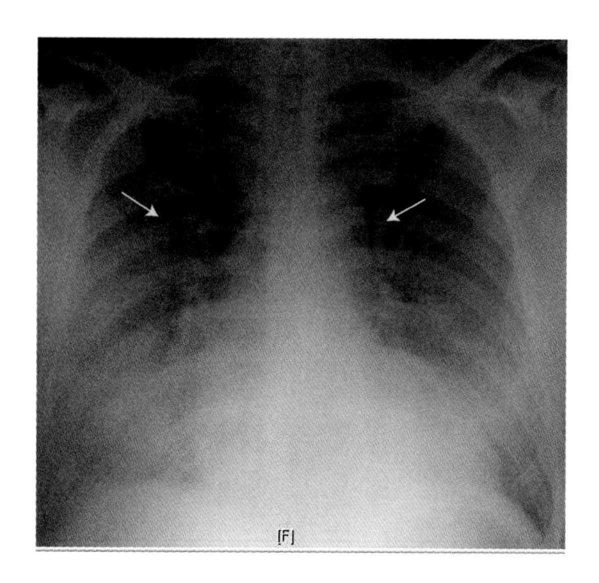

**Vessels are engorged with fluid in this patient with pulmonary edema.**

In cases where the history, physical, and x-ray are not clear, BNP is useful for diagnosing CHF. A normal BNP will exclude pulmonary edema. Also, troponin/CK-MB test should be done.

**Chemistry:** There are 2 ways to get tests. One way is to "get a bunch of tests and let's see what's there." The other way is to say, "If this is CHF, the BUN will be high and the sodium will be low. I am getting a BUN and sodium level to prove or disprove whether what I EXPECT to find is there."

- BUN:creatinine ratio >20:1 from pre-renal azotemia
- Hyponatremia is common.
- Hypokalemia and metabolic alkalosis is caused by chronic diuretic use.

Echocardiogram is not needed in acute management because it does not change management. Initial therapy is not altered whether it is systolic or diastolic dysfunction. An echo should be ordered but it is not urgent. The most important use of echo is in determining choice of medication for long-term use if the diagnosis of CHF is not clear.

## Treatment

- Administer oxygen and elevate head of bed
- Furosemide (Lasix) IV every 20–30 minutes until urine is produced
  - If no furosemide has been used, start with 10 mg, then 20 mg, then 40 mg, then 80 mg given via IV push.
  - If furosemide was previously being used, start with an IV version of the patient's usual dose. If patient had taken 40 mg bid, then give 40 IV, then 80 mg, then 160 mg every 20–30 minutes until urine is produced.
- Strict monitoring of intake and output ("I & O") to be sure there has been a response
- Nitroglycerin: paste, IV, or sublingual
- Morphine 2–4 mg IV

Refractory cases of pulmonary edema will need to be treated with hemodialysis. If the fluid will not come off any other way, then take it off with dialysis.

### Who should be sent to the ICU?

- Those where oxygen, diuretics, nitrates, and morphine do not control the dyspnea
- Those with systolic BP (SBP) <90 mmHg, making the use of diuretics difficult
- Those with acute MI or ventricular arrhythmia

**Round Saver**

Do not use beta blockers in acutely ill patients.

For **ICU management**, do not stop oxygen, diuretics, or nitrates. ICU management of pulmonary edema is extremely variable between institutions. The following treatments have no clear mortality benefit, thus decisions about which ones to pursue will vary with each attending physician.

Consider adding the following to treatment:

- Positive inotropes: dobutamine, imamrinone, or milrinone
- Sick enough for ICU = cardiology consult
- Treat MI or arrhythmia if present
- CPAP/BiPAP
- Nesiritide (IV atrial natriuretic peptide)

Intubate if hypoxia persists despite these treatments.

**For management in the clinic**, the No. 1 complaint is **shortness of breath**. Patients do not present in clinic with the obvious rales, gallop, tachycardia, abnormal ABG, and chest x-ray that they do in the hospital. The diagnosis is based on:

**Dyspnea +/– peripheral edema +/– rales**

## Diagnostic Testing

The most important test is an echo. This is the only way to be sure of:

- Ejection fraction
- Systolic vs. diastolic dysfunction
- Valvular function

EKG, chemistries, and chest x-ray should also be performed in all patients. The most important findings on EKG are:

- Q waves: sign of old infarction
- Left ventricular hypertrophy: S wave in V1 and R wave in V5 >35 mm
- Atrial fibrillation or flutter

## Treatment

The best initial therapy is based on whether there is systolic or diastolic dysfunction. You can only determine this from the echo. Systolic dysfunction is often used interchangeably with the term dilated cardiomyopathy. The ejection fraction (EF) is low (<40%). The heart in systolic dysfunction can relax, but cannot contract. In diastolic dysfunction, the opposite is true. The ejection fraction is preserved at normal. The heart can contract normally, but cannot relax.

### Systolic Dysfunction

- ACE inhibitors: All are equal in efficacy in the class. Angiotensin receptor blockers (ARBs) are an alternative to ACE inhibitors. The No. 1 use for ARBs is treatment of cough from ACE inhibitors.
- Beta blockers: metoprolol, carvedilol, bisoprolol
- Spironolactone: Used only in advanced stage class III or IV CHF. Class III/IV CHF is when there are symptoms with minimum exertion or at rest. Spironolactone causes gynecomastia; for those cases eplerenone is the alternative to spironolactone.
- Diuretics and digoxin are used in CHF but are not clearly associated with a mortality benefit. Diuretics are used in anyone with fluid overload. Digoxin decreases symptoms only in those still feeling ill despite the other therapies.
- Biventricular pacemaker lowers more mortality if there is systolic dysfunction and there is a QRS >120 msec. This "resynchronizes" the ventricles so they beat more efficiently together.
- Automatic implantable cardioverter defibrillator (AICD): Lowers mortality in those with persistently low EF despite maximal medical therapy.
- Hydralazine and nitrate combination: Used as an alternative therapy in those unable to take ACEIs or ARBs, particularly those with persistent hyperkalemia.

### Diastolic Dysfunction

There are no medications or devices proven to clearly lower mortality in patients with diastolic dysfunction. The presentation and testing of diastolic dysfunction is identical to systolic dysfunction. Although there are no medications clearly proven to lower mortality, the standard of care is to use:

- Beta blockers: metoprolol, carvedilol, bisoprolol
- Diuretics
- ACE inhibitors are not clearly beneficial

## Hypertensive Crisis (Emergency)

Hypertensive crisis is defined as severe hypertension with end-organ damage such as:

- CNS: confusion
- Heart: chest pain
- Lung: dyspnea or CHF
- Eye: blurry vision
- Renal insufficiency

### Treatment

Treatment is any IV antihypertensive medication such as labetalol, enalaprilat, or nitroprusside. Do not lower the blood pressure >25% in the first few hours so a stroke doesn't occur.

## Cardiomyopathy

Cardiomyopathy is defined as any cardiac muscular disorder that impairs the function of either contraction or relaxation. The ejection fraction can be high or low. In all cases, the patient feels short of breath, which worsens on exertion and improves with rest. There are usually rales on examination and can be peripheral edema.

## Diagnostic Testing

Chest x-ray can show congestion or pulmonary vascular redistribution, and the most noninvasive test is an echo.

There are 2 tests that technically are more accurate for the ejection fraction:

- Nuclear ventriculogram (MUGA)
- Left heart cardiac catheterization

Neither of these tests is routinely done, but they are more accurate than an echo.

**Systolic dysfunction = dilated cardiomyopathy = relaxes OK/contraction bad**

**Diastolic dysfunction = hypertrophic cardiomyopathy = contracts OK/relaxation bad**

Restrictive cardiomyopathy neither contracts nor relaxes well. The infiltrative diseases that cause it make the myocardium immobile. Restrictive cardiomyopathy is caused by:

- Sarcoidosis
- Amyloidosis
- Hemochromatosis
- Cancer
- Endomyocardial fibrosis

## Treatment

Dilated cardiomyopathy (same treatment as systolic dysfunction):

- Beta blockers

- ACE inhibitors or ARBs (hydralazine and nitrates are alternatives)
- Spironolactone or eplerenone
- Diuretics

**Round Saver** 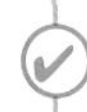

Hydralazine is an alternative to ACEs and ARBs

Hypertrophic cardiomyopathy (same treatment as diastolic dysfunction):

- Beta blockers
- Diuretics

Restrictive cardiomyopathy:

- Correct the underlying cause

## Hypertrophic Obstructive Cardiomyopathy (HOCM)

HOCM is an idiopathic disorder with an abnormal shape to the septum of the heart that leads to a physical obstruction to the outflow tract of blood. Similar to hypertrophic cardiomyopathy is the preservation of ejection fraction and the use of beta blockers. Anything that empties the ventricle increases the outflow tract obstruction. The main difference is:

HOCM is associated with syncope and, rarely, sudden death in healthy young athletes.

**Things You Will Be Asked on Rounds**

- Episodes of lightheadedness
- Loss of consciousness
- Chest pain
- Previous echo or EKG

## Physical Findings

- S4 gallop
- Systolic murmur: crescendo/decrescendo at lower left sternal border (LLSB)
- Murmur
  - Valsalva and standing: WORSE (louder)
- Squatting and leg raise: BETTER (softer)

## Diagnostic Testing

The initial test is an echo. EKG will show left ventricular hypertrophy. The most accurate test is left heart catheterization.

## Treatment

- Beta blocker (metoprolol) (first therapy)
- Implantable defibrillator (for syncope)

Round Saver 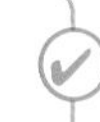

Diuretics, ACEIs, ARBs, dehydration, and digoxin will worsen HOCM.

# ARRHYTHMIAS

The most important issue for anyone admitted with an arrhythmia is **hemodynamic stability**. Hemodynamic instability is defined as:

- Hypotensive (systolic blood pressure <90 mmHg)
- Shortness of breath (dyspnea)
- Altered mental status/confusion for inadequate perfusion
- Chest pain

For anyone who is hemodynamically unstable:

- Call your resident if you are the first person to find it.
- Recheck the blood pressure.
- Normal saline is required.
- Repeat EKG.

As a new student on the Wards for your Medicine rotation, you have no "experiential base" to determine who is extremely ill from who can wait. A hemodynamically unstable arrhythmia of any kind as defined as chest pain, shortness of breath, hypotension, or confusion moves immediately to the top of the "most dangerous" list.

### Palpitations

Palpitations are very nonspecific. The patient has no disease at all 50% of the time. You must do an EKG.

1. If EKG is normal, do a Holter monitor as an outpatient or telemetry as an inpatient.
2. Do not overtreat. If there is no objective pathology found, do not medicate.
3. Exclude thyroid disease, alcohol excess or excess caffeine use.

## Atrial Fibrillation and Flutter

Atrial fibrillation (A-fib) and atrial flutter (Aflut) are addressed as if they are one disease because the testing and treatment are essentially the same. Patients with A-fib do not present saying, "I am here because of my long-standing hypertension and dilated left atrium." A-fib and Aflut present with:

- Palpitations or fluttering in the chest
- Lightheadedness
- "Racing" heart
- Loss of consciousness is rare, but possible
- Chest pain in some

### Things You Will Be Asked on Rounds

- Hypertension (most common)
- CHF or cardiomyopathy of any kind
- Thyroid disease
- Alcohol or cocaine use (alcohol definitely causes transient episodes of A-fib)
- Rheumatic fever, particularly in immigrants
- Previous EKG/Holter monitor/echo

## Physical Findings

The most important feature of A-fib, by far, is an irregularly irregular heart rhythm.

Do not measure the heart rate by palpating the radial pulse. All beats are not transmitted sufficiently and may not be felt at the radial pulse because the heart is only partially full during a number of the beats. You must have a systolic BP of ≥90/min to feel a radial pulse. Weak contractions will not transmit.

## Diagnostic Testing

**EKG**: absence of P wave, QRS <100 mSec (normal), irregularly irregular as based on R-to-R intervals

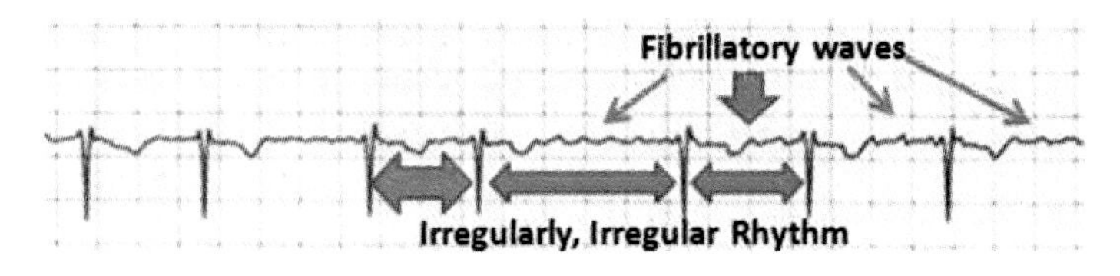


**P-waves are absent; fibrillatory waves and the R-to-R intervals are irregularly irregular, with no fixed pattern.**

**Holter monitor:** ambulatory patients

**Telemetry:** inpatients

**CK-MB and troponin:** patients with acute episodes of rapid rate

**Echocardiography:** everyone, if not done in last 6 months

Echo is indispensible for detecting valve disease, which may have led to A-fib/Aflut. Echo is essential to look at valve function and for clots. Clots need anticoagulation. Valvular disease leading to A-fib/Aflut needs warfarin in many cases.

**Stress test:** sometimes useful

Ischemia is not a frequent direct cause of atrial arrhythmia. In general, atrial arrhythmia is caused by a dilated atrium.

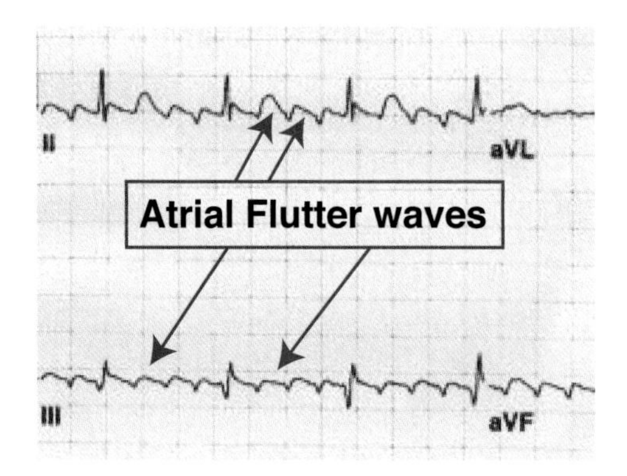


**Flutter waves are regular and uniform, with normal QRS (<100 mSec).**

## Treatment

Slowing the rate is usually the first step in the management of A-fib/Aflut. The goal is heart rate <100–110/min. The 2 best therapies are:

- Metoprolol: 5 mg IV every 5 minutes for 3 doses. Then start oral 50 mg bid. Maximum 200 bid.
- Diltiazem: 0.25 mg/kg with a second IV dose of 0.35 mg/kg. Then start oral 30 mg qid. Maximum 120 qid.

Both metoprolol and diltiazem should control the rate within 30 minutes. If one of these does not work and systolic BP is >90–100 mmHg, you can add the other.

If BP is low or borderline, use digoxin. Digoxin is not a first choice in stable patients because it is not great at controlling the heart rate on exertion. In hospital settings, however, when A-fib/Aflut is rapid and BP low, digoxin is very useful. Digoxin is slower than calcium blockers or beta blockers but will not lower BP. In fact, when the heart rate is controlled, it can raise the BP.

- Digoxin: 0.25 mg IV every 2 hours. Orally every 6 hours. Most patients are controlled with 1–1.5 mg. Digoxin does not lower the blood pressure like beta blockers or calcium channel blockers.

Other medications for rate control of rapid atrial arrhythmias are:

- Verapamil
- Beta blockers: esmolol, propranolol, atenolol

**Round Saver**

Know the maximum dose of every drug you use.

## Rate Control vs. Rhythm Control

Routine cardioversion to sinus rhythm is not correct. It is correct to slow the rate with beta blockers, calcium blockers, and occasionally digoxin. Cardioversion is done urgently in the occasional case that is hemodynamically unstable. Most patients will not stay in sinus rhythm if you use medications such as amiodarone, procainamide, propafenone or dofetilide to convert them. In addition, these medications can cause arrhythmias such as Torsade de pointes. This is particularly true of dofetilide and ibutilide.

Electrical cardioversion for hemodynamically stable patients needs a TEE beforehand to make sure there is no clot and for anticoagulation with warfarin for 3–4 weeks afterward. Cardioversion is only occasionally performed for atrial fibrillation after rate control if the patient is young and has an otherwise anatomically normal heart. If there is a dilated left atrium or significant valve disease, the patient simply will not stay in sinus rhythm.

**Anticoagulation** is not indicated if the arrhythmia has been present for <48 hours. Anticoagulate if there is significant risk for a stroke.

Risk factors for stroke are the following, summarized as **CHADS**:

- Dilated **C**ardiomyopathy (1 point)
- **H**ypertension (1 point)
- Older **A**ge, particularly >75 (1 point)
- **D**iabetes mellitus (1 point)
- Prior **S**troke or TIA is a clear indication for anticoagulation (2 points for either one)

Each of these factors is assigned 1 point, except for stroke or TIA, which gets 2 points. This is so that anyone with a previous stroke or TIA will automatically be started on anticoagulation.

- When CHADS score is **0 or 1**: aspirin or aspirin and clopidogrel (The use of aspirin for CHADS 0 or 1 is controversial at this time. Find out the preferences of your attending physician.)
- When CHADS is **2 or more**: anticoagulation with warfarin, rivaroxaban, or dabigatran

Warfarin is difficult to use. Maintaining an INR of 2–3 is problematic and it takes several days to achieve. There is no need for routine "bridging therapy" with heparin every time you use warfarin. Heparin causes bleeding and thrombocytopenia. Even with waiting several days for warfarin to become therapeutic, you do not need to use heparin if the reason for the warfarin is only A-fib. Use heparin if a clot is present.

Rivaroxaban and dabigatran:

- No INR monitoring necessary
- Therapeutic on the same day you start
- No treatment to reverse them if patient bleeds
- At least as effective or even better than warfarin

## Supraventricular Tachycardia (SVT)

SVT presents with the sudden onset of palpitations or a "racing heart" that may lead to shortness of breath. Heart rate is approximately 160/min and there are no specific physical findings. Ischemia is rarely a cause of SVT so if the patient presents with an acute MI as the cause of palpitations, you should question whether SVT is causing the symptoms. SVT is most often caused by an abnormal conduction pathway around the AV node.

**Things You Will Be Asked on Rounds**

SVT Characteristics

- Palpitations
- Lightheadedness
- Speed of onset of symptoms

### Diagnostic Testing

SVT is an EKG diagnosis. EKG will show a rapid, narrow complex (<100 msec) tachycardia, usually at a rate of 160/min. P wave, fibrillatory waves, and flutter waves are not visible.

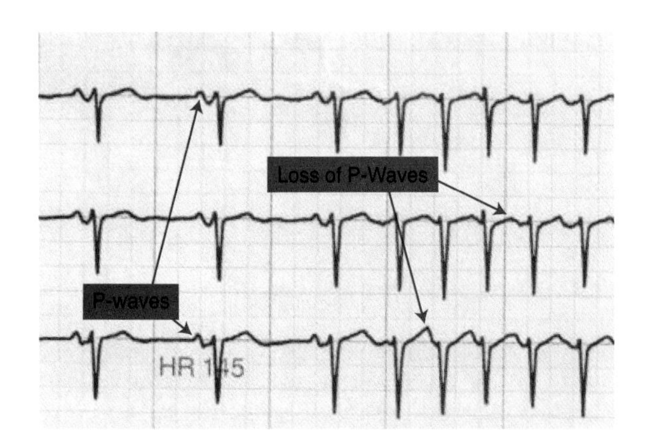


**Notice the loss of P-wave and speeding of rate; there are no flutter waves, P-waves, or fibrillatory waves.**

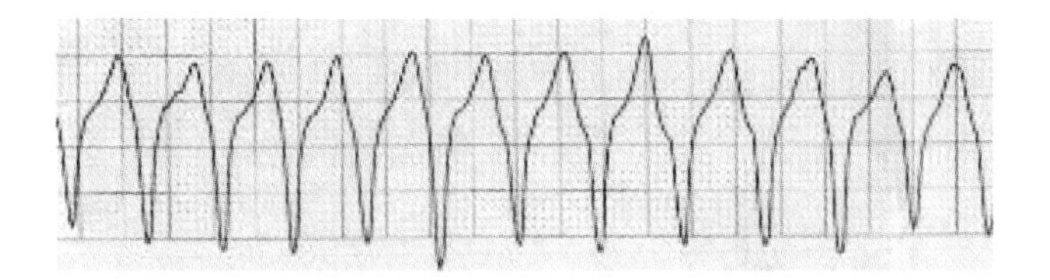

**Classic example of wide complex tachycardia**

Telemetry monitoring should be used in all patients with SVT. Echocardiography shows nothing specific in SVT but should be done to exclude other pathology.

CK-MB and troponin levels have little use. Your house staff and attending physician will always state this, yet patients admitted with SVT always seem to have cardiac enzyme tests done.

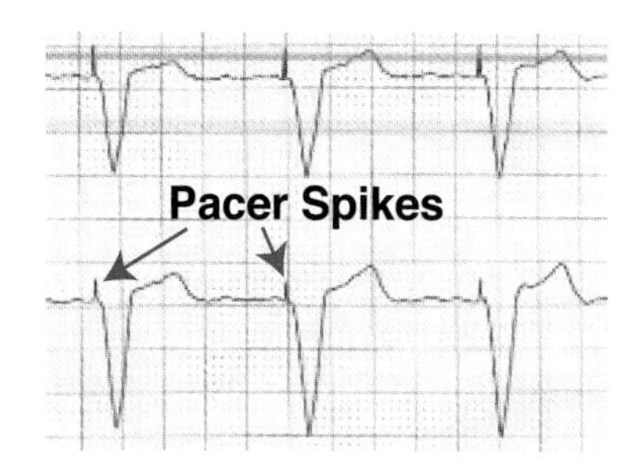


**A single-chamber pacemaker in the ventricle. Note the sharp, vertical pacer spike. Conduction is slow and wide because it is not going through the normal, rapid conduction system.**

### Treatment

- Vagal maneuvers: carotid massage, Valsalva maneuver, gagging, and diving reflex
- Adenosine
- Metoprolol or diltiazem
- Electrical cardioversion (for rare cases of hemodynamically unstable or nonresponse to other therapies)

## Wolff-Parkinson-White Syndrome (WPW)

WPW presents with:

- Supraventricular tachycardia (SVT)
- SVT alternating with ventricular tachycardia
- Delta wave found on EKG done for other purposes

Look for a patient with palpitations, lightheadedness, or occasionally syncope.

### Things You Will Be Asked on Rounds

- Previous EKG
- Worsening symptoms or arrhythmia with the use of digoxin or calcium channel blockers
- Previous catheterization or electrophysiology studies

## Diagnostic Testing

EKG will show short PR (normal 120–200 msec) and delta waves from early depolarization of the ventricle.

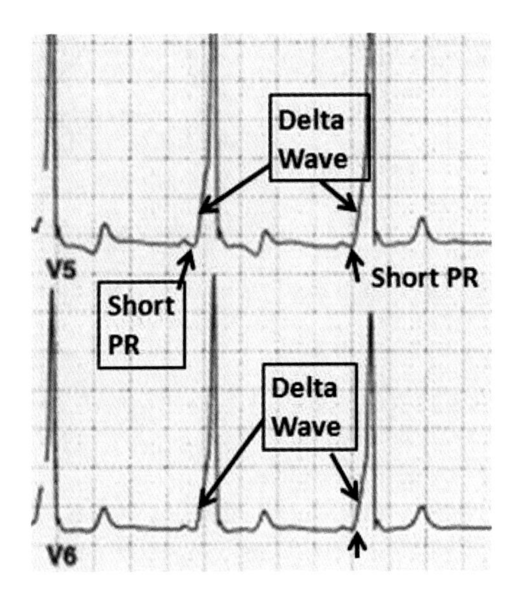


**WPW has short PR interval (<120 mSec) and a delta wave indicative of abnormal early depolarization of the ventricle.**

Electrophysiology (EP) study is the most accurate test, done by placing a catheter into the heart and electrically testing the cardiac circuits. EP study is the only way to know the exact electrical circuitry of the heart.

### Treatment

- Procainamide, amiodarone, flecainide, or sotalol (for SVT or ventricular tachycardia that is occurring at the moment)
- Ablation (permanent cure)

The majority of patients with WPW come to the hospital with palpitations or with a delta wave and short PR found on an EKG done for other reasons. Most are not having an arrhythmia at the present moment. In those cases, refer for electrophysiology (EP) study to identify the abnormal conduction tract. Eliminate that tract immediately with ablation or "electrocautery" of the abnormal tract.

## Multifocal Atrial Tachycardia (MAT)

MAT is an atrial arrhythmia found in association with COPD. MAT has 3 P-wave morphologies and a normal width of QRS (100 msec).

Treatment is the same as for A-fib and Aflut. Beta blockers are avoided because of their potential to worsen COPD.

## Ventricular Tachycardia (VT)

VT is always considered an extreme emergency. Any sustained ventricular tachycardia needs the following rapid response:

- Immediately call your resident.
- Check blood pressure.

- If systolic BP <90 mmHg, give bolus of saline and activate "code" for emergency response.
- Hook up continuous EKG.
- Check for chest pain, confusion, or shortness of breath.
- Get a cardioverter/defibrillator INTO THE ROOM in case you need it.

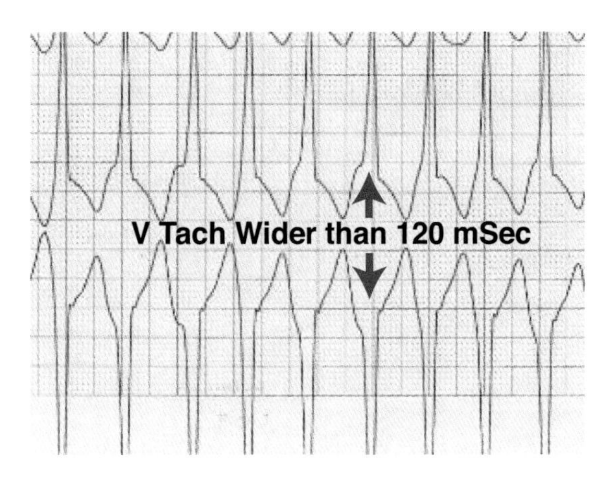


**While normal QRS is usually <100 mSec, in ventricular tachycardia it is usually wider than 120 mSec and reproducibly regular.**

With presentation, short "runs" of VT of 5 or 10 seconds are not defined precisely as "sustained." Sustained VT has been defined at 30 seconds or more. However, these "nonsustained" runs of VT can occur in patients in the ICU, on telemetry, or in the emergency department with limited hemodynamic effects.

The most important issues regarding VT on the Wards are the following:

1. Is blood pressure normal? (SBP >90–100 mmHg)
2. Are the brain, heart, and lungs being perfused?
3. Is the VT continuing?

## Things You Will Be Asked on Rounds

- Previous history of an MI (ischemia is the most common reason for VT)
- CK-MB and troponin levels
- Potassium, magnesium, calcium, and oxygen levels
- Medications patient is on
- Has an echocardiogram been done?

All antiarrhythmic medication except beta blockers can potentially cause arrhythmias. Low levels of magnesium, calcium, and oxygen cause ventricular arrhythmias. High or low potassium levels cause arrhythmias. Cocaine intoxication can cause arrhythmias. All cardiomyopathies, especially dilated cardiomyopathy with a low ejection fraction can cause ventricular arrhythmias.

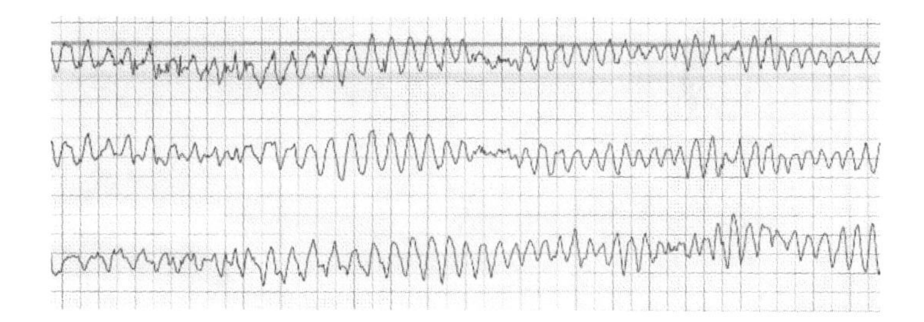

**Torsade is ventricular tachycardia with undulating amplitude.**

### Treatment

Unstable patients need immediate synchronized cardioversion. Unstable is defined as:

- Systolic BP <90 mmHg
- Chest pain
- Shortness of breath
- Confusion from decreased cerebral perfusion

Stable patients are treated with magnesium and medications such as:

- Amiodarone
- Lidocaine
- Procainamide

## Ventricular Fibrillation

All patients with ventricular fibrillation need to have cardiopulmonary resuscitation (CPR) started immediately followed by an unsynchronized cardioversion. CPR basically means chest compressions at a rate of 100/minute and respirations. There should be 2 ventilations for every 30 compressions, or ratio 30:2. If there is no response to CPR and defibrillation, give epinephrine or vasopressin and shock the patient again while trying to do CPR continuously except for the very moment the electricity is given.

**Ventricular fibrillation = CPR + electrical shock**

Amiodarone is preferred over lidocaine. Lidocaine is only used if amiodarone is not available. Ventricular tachycardia without a pulse is treated the same way as ventricular fibrillation.

For ventricular fibrillation, the plan is:

1. CPR
2. Shock (unsynchronized cardioversion = defibrillation)
3. CPR
4. Epinephrine (or vasopressin)
5. Continue CPR
6. Shock again 2 minutes after the first shock
7. Continue CPR
8. Amiodarone

## Bradycardia

The most important issue with bradycardia is whether the patient is hemodynamically stable or unstable. Although a normal pulse is 60–100/min, many people can have a pulse <60 but with no symptoms. If the patient has bradycardia with no symptoms, perform an EKG to determine the etiology. Sinus bradycardia, first-degree AV block, and Mobitz type I (Wenckebach) require no treatment if they are asymptomatic. Mobitz II and third-degree AV (complete) heart block require a pacemaker even if they are asymptomatic.

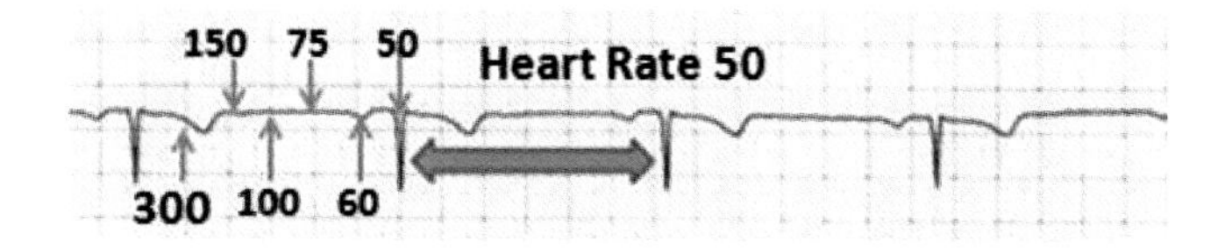


**Each large box is 200 milliseconds. More than 5 large boxes between beats indicates bradycardia.**

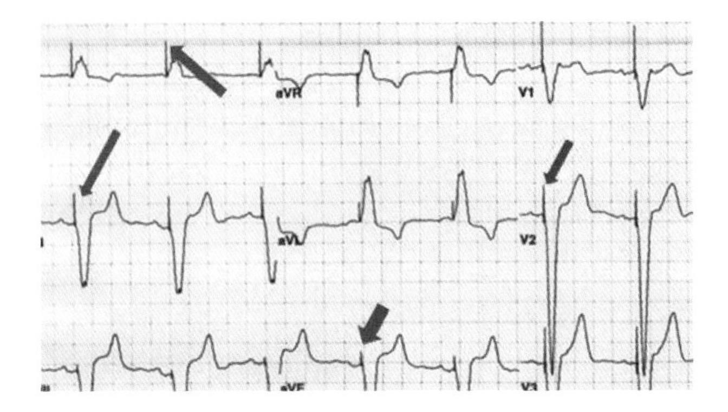


**Sharp vertical pacer spikes (under arrows) from a single chamber ventricular pacemaker give a wide complex QRS and abnormal T-wave which make interpretation for ischemia nearly impossible.**

## Things You Will Be Asked on Rounds

- Low blood pressure (systolic <90 mmHg)
- Lightheadedness
- Confusion or disorientation
- Syncope
- Shortness of breath

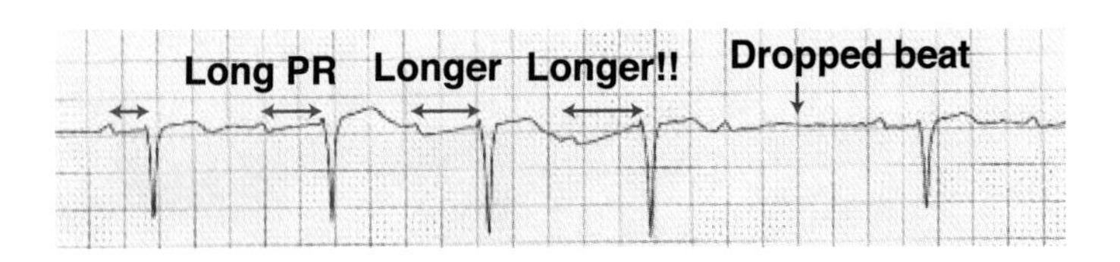


**PR interval gradually prolongs from beat to beat; then a QRS is dropped.**

### Treatment

Unstable bradycardia of any etiology

- Atropine 0.5–1.0 mg IV immediately (maximum 3 mg)
- Transcutaneous pacemaker
- Permanent transvenous pacemaker

> **Round Saver**
>
> Mobitz I: no treatment
>
> Mobitz II: pacemaker

Do not get tortured by people leading you away from using atropine for symptomatic bradycardia. Just because it does not work in everyone does not mean you should not try it.

Stable bradycardia (asymptomatic)

- Sinus, first-degree AV block, and Mobitz I: no treatment
- Mobitz II second-degree AV block and third-degree (complete) heart block: pacemaker

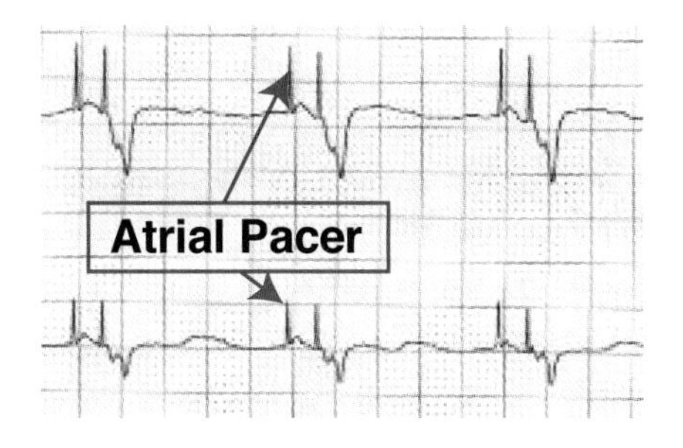


**The first pacer spike triggers the atrium; the second triggers the ventricle.**

## Sick Sinus Syndrome

This is also known as "tachy-brady syndrome," in which there is an alternating fast and slow heart rate. Patients will need:

- Pacemaker if too slow (e.g., pause >3 seconds)
- Beta blockers if too fast

1. Basic life support (BLS) on frequency of compressions and ventilations
2. Advanced cardiac life support (ACLS) on cardiac arrest
3. ACLS on bradycardia with pulse

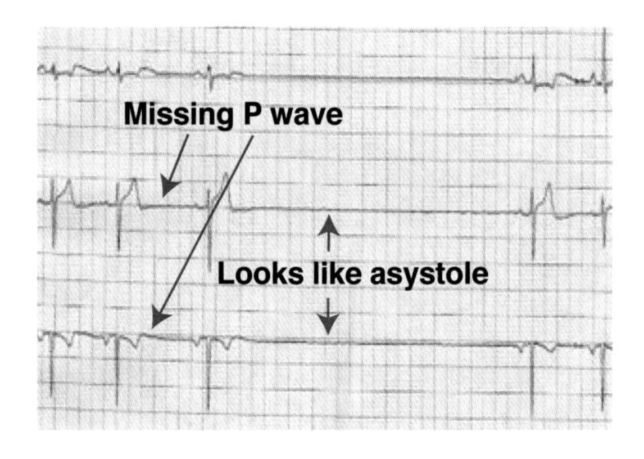


**P-waves simply stop occurring. The middle part looks like asystole, but P-waves restart spontaneously.**

## Syncope

The most important issue in syncope is to exclude the cardiac and neurologic causes of syncope. 80–90% of the mortality is with syncope from a cardiac or neurologic etiology. The most dangerous causes of syncope are:

- Myocardial infarction
- Ventricular arrhythmia
- Aortic stenosis
- HOCM

- Seizure
- Brainstem stroke

## Diagnostic Testing

Despite a history and physical, nearly everyone with syncope gets the same in-hospital evaluation. The tests for syncope are:

- EKG
- CK-MB and troponin
- Telemetry monitor (Holter in outpatients)
- Echocardiogram
- Oxygen, glucose, sodium, and calcium level

If you order all of these tests whether you understand the case or not, you will likely arrive at the right diagnosis of syncope (i.e., you will detect any dangerous pathology). In most patients, the cause of syncope will not be found.

With syncope, your job is to exclude dangerous pathology such as MI or arrhythmia. On the Wards, this role is different from the role you have with other cardiac disease. In other diseases, you must find the cause and the definite treatment. So many people admitted with syncope do not in fact have syncope, or they have such benign causes of it (e.g., a vasovagal episode) that your endpoint is different. Again, it is not your job to find a definite cause, but rather to find something that could be dangerous (e.g., MI, arrhythmia, or seizure).

### Things You Will Be Asked on Rounds

- Whether loss of consciousness was sudden or gradual
- Whether recovery of consciousness was sudden or gradual
- Presence of murmurs on examination

| Investigating Syncope | |
|---|---|
| ***Sudden*** loss of consciousness | Cardiac & neurologic causes (e.g., MI or seizure) |
| ***Gradual*** loss of consciousness | Toxi-metabolic causes: low glucose, hypoxia, drug overdose |
| **Sudden regaining** of consciousness | Cardiac: arrhythmia, MI, HOCM, or aortic stenosis (AS) |
| **Gradual regaining** of consciousness | Seizures, glucose, oxygen, and drug overdose |
| Murmur present | AS, mitral stenosis, HOCM |

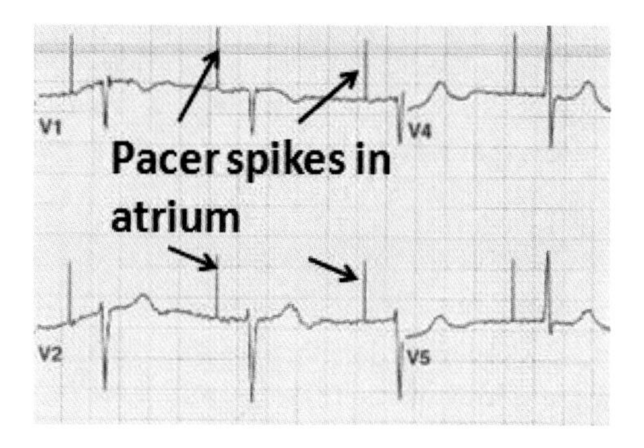


**Sharp vertical atrial pacer spikes are visible before QRS; after AV node, impulses go down normal conduction system resulting in fast, narrow QRS.**

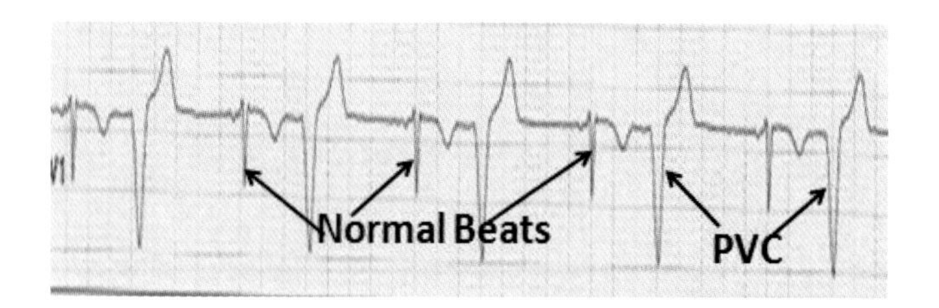


**Every other beat is a premature ventricular contraction (PVC); normal beats are narrow (QRS <100 mSec) and PVCs are wide. Bigeminy needs no specific treatment.**

### Common Errors in Syncope Diagnosis

- Carotid disease does not cause syncope, so carotid Dopplers are useless.
- Brainstem lesions causing syncope cannot be seen with a head CT. If you want to look at the brainstem, get an MRI. Head CT is useless for syncope caused by brainstem lesions.
- Getting an EEG in all syncope patients is extremely low yield.
- If there is a cardiac lesion severe enough to cause syncope, you will hear it on exam. An echo to evaluate for cardiac lesions in the absence of a murmur is extremely low yield. An echo for syncope without hearing a murmur is very unlikely to help you.

## VALVULAR HEART DISEASE

What can all forms of valvular heart disease have in common?

- Dyspnea
- CHF
- Edema
- Murmurs
- Congenital or caused by rheumatic fever

For valvular heart disease, echo is the best initial test. Catheterization, though rarely needed, is the most accurate test.

Endocarditis prophylaxis is never indicated unless the valve has been replaced.

Auscultation is extremely difficult to learn. You must always auscultate your patient's heart but you will need to ask for confirmation of what you find. The echo is so readily available that it has nearly killed auscultation.

Increased venous return increases the loudness and intensity of all murmurs except mitral valve prolapse (MVP) and HOCM.

Raising the patient's legs in the air passively or asking the patient to squat from a standing position increases venous return.

Decreased venous return does the opposite. Standing suddenly from a squatting position or Valsalva will decrease venous return. Standing and Valsalva decrease the intensity or loudness of all left-sided murmurs except for MVP.

Handgrip increases afterload. Handgrip is performed by auscultating the patient's heart while he or she squeezes your hand or a towel at the same time. This compresses the arteries of the arm and will increase the afterload. Handgrip will worsen regurgitant lesions such as aortic or mitral regurgitation. Handgrip may improve HOCM by keeping more blood in the heart and decreasing the outflow tract obstruction.

| Maneuver | Effect | Lesions Made Louder |
|---|---|---|
| Squatting, leg raise | Increases venous return | AR, MR, AS, MS |
| Standing, Valsalva | Decreases venous return | MVP, HOCM |
| Handgrip | Increases afterload | AR, MR |

## Aortic Regurgitation (AR) and Mitral Regurgitation (MR)

Both forms are common lesions that can occur from any cause of dilated cardiomyopathy. As the heart dilates up in size, the valve leaflets must separate.

**Cardiac dilation = regurgitation**

Other causes of regurgitant heart lesions are:

- Hypertension
- Myocardial infarction
- Endocarditis
- Myxomatous degeneration
- Rare: Marfan's, Ehlers-Danlos syndrome, ankylosing spondylitis

Many people diagnosed with AR and MR can be asymptomatic for many years. When symptomatic, patients present with dyspnea, rales, and edema. It is very difficult to distinguish a dilated cardiomyopathy that leads to AR and MR from AR and MR that led to a dilated cardiomyopathy. The presentation of regurgitant lesions is largely the same as that of dilated cardiomyopathy.

With AR, the **diastolic decrescendo murmur** is greatest at the lower left sternal border. With MR, the pansystolic or holosystolic murmur is heard best at the axilla and radiates to the axilla.

Both AR and MR murmurs become louder with leg raise and squatting, and softer with Valsalva and standing. Handgrip makes them worse; because handgrip increases afterload, AR and MR get worse because they are treated with ACE inhibitors and ARBs, which decrease afterload.

## Diagnostic Testing

Echo is the best test. With EKG, AR will show left ventricular hypertrophy (LVH).

**SV1 + RV5 >35 mm = LVH**

Chest x-ray will show enlarged left atrium (LA) and left ventricle (LV).

### Treatment

Initial therapy is ACE inhibitors (ACEIs). With intolerance of ACEIs (cough), use ARBs or nifedipine.

Neither AR nor MR needs antibiotic prophylaxis before a dental procedure unless the valve has been replaced.

Surgery is indicated to repair or replace the valve when the ejection fraction drops or the left ventricular end-systolic diameter increases. Repair is a surgical "tightening" of the valve by placing sutures into the ends of the valve to decrease its "leakiness."

**Indications for Surgical Repair**

| Lesion | Ejection Fraction | Left Ventricular End-Systolic Diameter |
|---|---|---|
| Aortic regurgitation | <50–55% | >50–55 mm |
| Mitral regurgitation | <60% | >45 mm |

## Aortic Stenosis (AS)

Aortic stenosis presents with:

- Angina (most common)
- Syncope
- CHF (worst prognosis)

It is associated with angina so frequently because (1) coronary artery disease (CAD) is so common in patients with AS, and (2) the stenotic aortic valve is in the way of physically perfusing the coronary arteries.

### Diagnostic Testing

Echo is the mainstay of testing, as it is in all valvular heart disease. EKG is done for severe LVH. Stress test and angiography are routinely done for AS because of the high frequency of CAD. Angiography is useful before surgical replacement of the valve because bypass surgery is frequently done at the same time.

### Treatment

Surgical replacement is required for all symptomatic patients. Balloon valvuloplasty is done instead when patients are too ill to undergo valve replacement

- ACE inhibitors and ARB do not help and can worsen symptoms
- Diuretics are sometimes useful in advanced disease with fluid overload. Patients with AS are very vulnerable to volume depletion.

Asymptomatic patients require no treatment.

## Mitral Stenosis

With mitral stenosis (MS), look for CHF. In addition, look for a young immigrant with:

- Dysphagia
- Hoarseness
- Atrial fibrillation
- Stroke at an early age

MS causes massive left atrial (LA) enlargement. This leads to atrial fibrillation and pressure on the esophagus and recurrent laryngeal nerve.

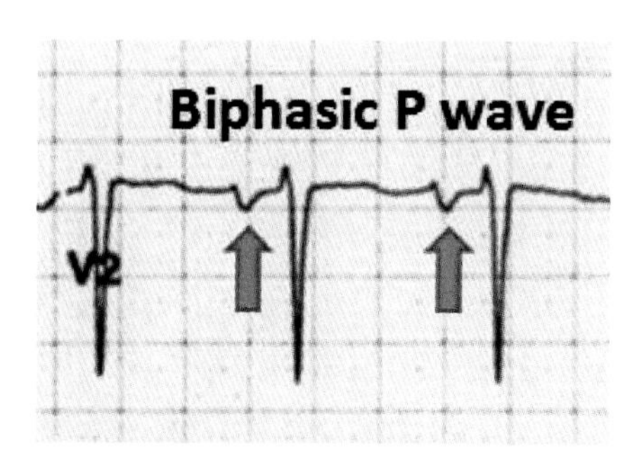


**Mitral stenosis causes left atrium to hypertrophy posteriorly and produce a biphasic P-wave in V1 and V2.**

## Diagnostic Testing

Transesophageal echo is best. EKG is done with biphasic P wave in V-1 and V-2 from left atrial hypertrophy. With chest x-ray, there is left atrial enlargement:

- "Double bubble" extra density behind the heart
- Pushing up the left mainstem bronchus
- Straightening of the left heart border

Left heart catheterization is the most accurate test.

## Treatment

- Diuretics control fluid overload
- Balloon valvuloplasty
- Digoxin or beta blockers only to control the heart rate with atrial arrhythmias
- Endocarditis prophylaxis is not necessary
- Valve replacement in those failing balloon dilation

# Mitral Valve Prolapse

Mitral valve prolapse (MVP) is an incidental finding of little significance. Most patients with MVP are asymptomatic and a click or murmur is found on routine examination. When it is occasionally symptomatic, MVP presents with:

- Palpitations
- Atypical chest pain (not related to exertion and not relieved by rest)

The **murmur** of MVP starts with a mid-systolic click followed by a late-systolic murmur of mitral regurgitation. This murmur will:

- Worsen with Valsalva and standing
- Improve with squatting or leg raising

This is because anything that empties the heart such as Valsalva or standing makes the heart smaller and exacerbates the click/murmur.

## Diagnostic Testing

Get an echo. The EKG and chest x-ray will be normal. Catheterization is not needed.

Treatment is beta blockers for palpitations and chest pain. Asymptomatic patients require no treatment or endocarditis prophylaxis.

# PERICARDIAL DISEASE

## Pericarditis

Acute pericarditis presents with chest pain that changes with position and with respiration. The pain is:

- Better when sitting up/worse when leaning back
- Worse usually on inspiration
- Associated with a friction rub on auscultation in 25–30% or less

**Things You Will Be Asked on Rounds**

- Fever and recent infection particularly of the lungs
- Renal failure
- Chest wall trauma
- Lupus and other collagen vascular disease such as rheumatoid arthritis or Wegener's
- Recent MI
- Cancer of organs in the chest

Pericarditis is caused by any infection, but viral infections are the most common.

### Diagnostic Testing

- EKG: ST-segment elevation in all leads except aVR
- PR-segment depression

### Treatment

Treat the underlying cause.

- NSAIDs such as ibuprofen and naproxen for most cases
  - Add colchicine to an NSAID to decrease risk of recurrence
- If an NSAID and colchicine do not control the symptoms, switch to a glucocorticoid such as prednisone

## Pericardial Tamponade

Tamponade is a hemodynamic disease that presents with shortness of breath and lightheadedness from hypotension. The patient will present with dyspnea. Look for:

- Hypotension
- Jugulovenous distention
- Tachycardia
- Pulsus paradoxus: a decrease in BP >10 mmHg with inhalation

Although tachycardia is extremely nonspecific, a normal heart rate strongly points away from pericardial tamponade.

### Things You Will Be Asked on Rounds

The causes of tamponade are the same infections, trauma, connective tissue disorders, and cancers that cause pericarditis.

- Fever and recent infection particularly of the lungs
- Renal failure
- Chest wall trauma
- Lupus and other collagen vascular disease such as rheumatoid arthritis or Wegener's
- Recent MI
- Cancer of organs in the chest

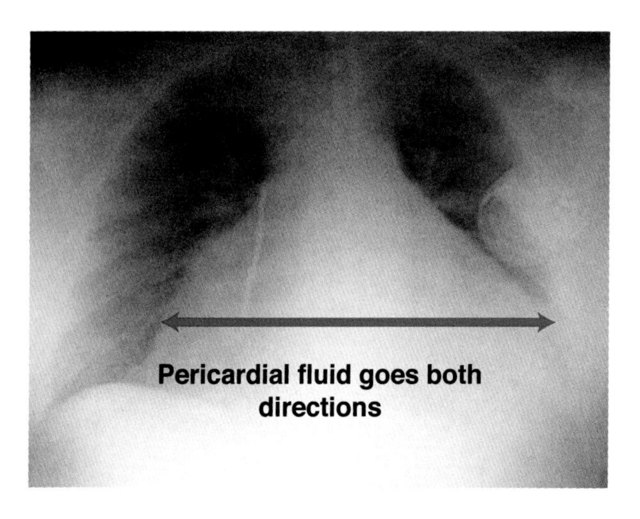


**Pericardial effusion enlarges the heart shadow both to the left and right.**

## Diagnostic Testing

An echo will show effusion pressing on the right side of the heart. Right atrial and right ventricular diastolic collapse is the first sign of tamponade

With EKG, low voltage will be present though nonspecific. Those who have COPD, are obese, or who have large breasts will also have low voltage. EKG will also show "electrical alternans," a variation in the height of the QRS complexes, which occur from the heart moving backward and forward in the chest.

With cardiac catheterization, there will be an equalization of pressure in all 4 chambers during diastole. This is rarely done but frequently asked about on rounds.

## Treatment

- Fluids help prevent/reverse tamponade
- Needle pericardiocentesis if tamponade is occurring
- Pericardial window placement

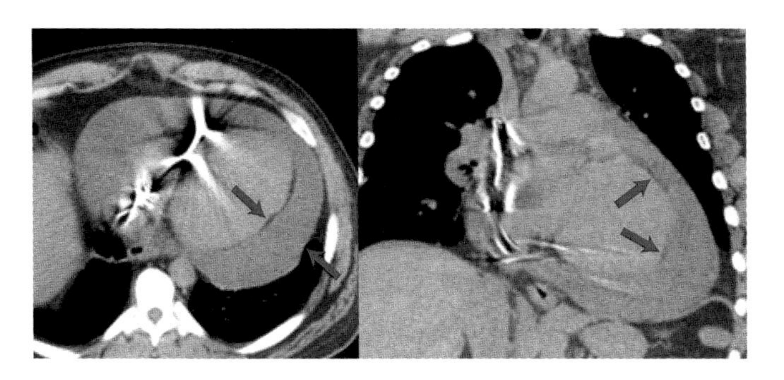

**Pericardial fluid is much more obvious on CT than echocardiogram, and CT is often faster to get.**

# Constrictive Pericarditis

Chronic pericardial infection or inflammation leads to chronic thickening, fibrosis, and calcification of the pericardium. This anatomic defect is associated with:

- Edema
- Jugulovenous distention
- Kussmaul's sign (increase in jugulovenous pressure on inhalation)
- Enlargement of the liver and spleen
- Ascites
- Pericardial "knock" as 3rd heart sound from filling of the ventricle hitting the fibrotic pericardium

### Diagnostic Testing

- Chest x-ray: fibrosis, thickening, and calcification of the pericardium
- Chest CT/MRI: shows the same as chest x-ray but in much greater detail
- Echo: less useful than it is in tamponade; fluid level is normal and the heart moves normally

Surgical removal is the only effective treatment. Although diuretics and salt restriction are used to prevent fluid buildup on the right side of the heart, the only meaningful management is to remove the pericardium.

## Peripheral Artery Disease (PAD)

PAD is angina of the calves. Look for:

- Pain in the legs relieved by rest
- Decreased peripheral pulses
- Smooth, shiny skin in severe cases

### Things You Will Be Asked on Rounds

- History of hypertension, diabetes, or hyperlipidemia
- History of tobacco smoking (extremely important)
- Does pain get better just by dangling legs over edge of bed?
- Pain with any exertion (spinal stenosis is worse walking downhill, not uphill)

## Diagnostic Testing

1. Ankle/brachial index (ABI)
2. Lower extremity Dopplers
3. Angiography

A normal person's ankle pressure will equal his arm (brachial) pressure when laying flat. When upright, ankle pressure is normally greater than arm, or brachial, pressure. If the ankle pressure >10%—lower than the brachial pressure (ABI <0.9)—there is an obstruction to the flow of blood in the legs.

## Treatment

The patient must stop smoking immediately and use:

- Aspirin (clopidogrel if aspirin not tolerated)
- Cilostazol
- ACE inhibitors for BP
- Statins to control LDL <100 mg/dL
- Tight control of glucose in diabetics

# AORTIC DISEASE

## Abdominal Aortic Disease

Screening for abdominal aortic aneurysm (AAA) should be done in all men age >65 who have ever smoked. It should be done with an ultrasound. If the AAA >5.0 cm, refer for surgical repair. If <5 cm, repeat the ultrasound in 6 months to look for an increase in diameter.

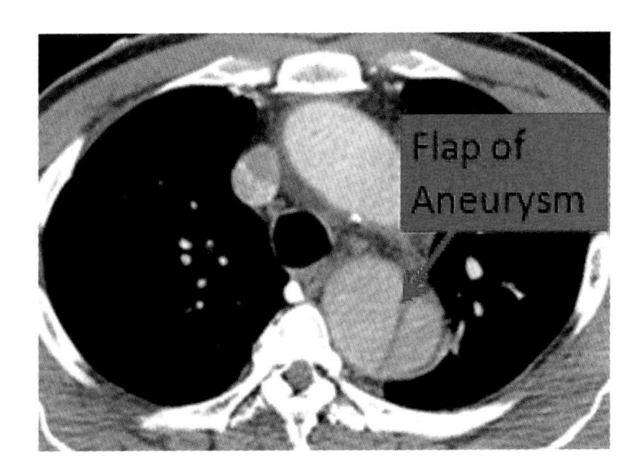


**Dissection is present with the torn flap of the aneurysm seen in the middle of a thoracic aneurysm.**

## Thoracic Aortic Aneurysm

There is no routine screening test for a thoracic aortic aneurysm. Patients present with:

- Chest pain
- Radiating straight through to the back
- Extremely severe cases have uneven pulses between arms
- Wide mediastinum on a chest x-ray.

## Diagnostic Testing

Whether or not the mediastinum is wide on the chest x-ray, the next best test is one of the following:

- CT angiogram
- Magnetic resonance angiography (MRA)
- Trans-esophageal echo (TEE)

Each of these tests has a 90–95% sensitivity and specificity. CT angiogram is used more often simply because an aortogram by CT is easy to obtain. The most accurate test is angiogram with a catheter but this is rarely needed.

Treatment is a beta blocker such as labetalol (to decrease pulse pressure), nitroprusside, or surgical repair.

# Pregnancy and Heart Disease

It is critical to know the most dangerous heart diseases to have during pregnancy. In order of the most dangerous first, they are:

1. Peripartum cardiomyopathy with persistent left ventricular dysfunction
2. Eisenmenger's phenomenon
3. Mitral stenosis
4. Aortic stenosis

Eisenmenger's phenomenon is a septal defect in the heart leading to pulmonary hypertension. When the left-to-right shunt becomes so severe that pulmonary hypertension develops, the patient starts to reverse into a right-to-left shunt. This means that any additional blood volume will be shunted directly from the right side of the heart to the left side. Right-to-left shunts are more dangerous than left-to-right shunts because the blood in right-to-left shunts bypasses the lungs and is not oxygenated.

In pregnancy, blood volume will increase by 50%. In Eisenmenger's, because there is severe pulmonary hypertension, all of the new blood volume will shunt directly into the left-sided circulation without being oxygenated.

# Endocrinology 2

## Diabetes Mellitus

The management of diabetes mellitus (DM) on your Wards rotation is markedly skewed toward the management of diabetic ketoacidosis (DKA) and very high glucose levels in general. This is because numerous illnesses present with hyperglycemia because of increased stress hormone production. Stress hormones are:

- Cortisol
- Catecholamines (norepinephrine and epinephrine)
- Glucagon
- Growth hormone

Remember that in adults, growth hormone is a "stress hormone" that raises glucose and free fatty acid levels. It does not normally cause "growth" in an adult.

**Round Saver**

Never show up to rounds without recent lab values.

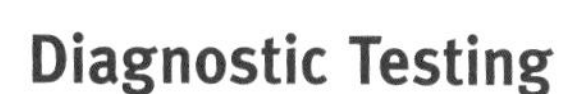

### Diagnostic Testing

The most important tests in acute cases of DM are the following:

- Serum bicarbonate and anion gap
- Glucose levels
- Potassium level
- Arterial (or venous) blood gas (ABG)

You may be surprised that the serum bicarbonate is put on top as the most important test. This is because your No. 1 issue for acute hyperglycemia is, "Is this patient acidotic?" Acidosis raises blood potassium level.

## Treatment

The presence of acidosis determines where in the hospital the patient should be managed. Acidotic patients go to the ICU. Acidosis is defined as:

- Low serum bicarbonate
- pH <7.3

ICU admission is not determined according to the glucose level. You can be acidotic with a glucose level of 200 or 300 mg/dL and need the ICU. You can have normal pH and bicarbonate and potassium levels with glucose of 500 mg/dL and safely place the patient on a general hospital ward.

**Round Saver**

Know the outpatient medications.

Severe acidosis needs IV insulin. If the pH <7.0–7.1, some attending physicians will give IV bicarbonate as well. The lower the pH and bicarbonate, the more severe the illness.

Death is near when:

- Bicarbonate <8–10 mEq/L
- pH <7.0
- Hyperkalemia >7 mEq/L

## Complications of DM

There are 2 serious conditions that patients with DM can develop: **diabetic ketoacidosis** and **nonketotic hyperosmolar syndrome**.

## Diabetic Ketoacidosis

Diabetic ketoacidosis (DKA) can occur with both types 1 and 2 diabetes. Although the classic answer is, "type 1 patients get DKA more often," there are 25 people with type 2 diabetes for every person with type 1, so on your rotation you may not see a preponderance of one type.

Look for a patient with:

- Hyperventilation from respiratory compensation for metabolic acidosis
- Confusion from a hyperosmolar state
- Generalized severe weakness from severe volume depletion
- Polyuria, polydipsia, and polyphagia

DKA is based on an insufficiency or resistance to insulin. If there isn't enough insulin, the cells can't pick up glucose. If there isn't enough glucose, the cells need to break down fat to "eat." Metabolized fat creates ketones which are partially digested "fat garbage." Ketones are enough to keep you alive, and the brain, with time, can switch to using them as a fuel source.

Ketones are acids, however, and bicarbonate gets used up to buffer them. The acid or hydrogen ion ($H^+$) is absorbed into the cells to "buffer" off the acid. Potassium ($K^+$) is released from cells in exchange to maintain electrical neutrality. One proton goes into the cell ($H^+$) and one proton ($K^+$) comes out of the cell. This creates hyperkalemia. The kidney excretes the potassium to prevent an arrhythmia. This leads to a loss of body potassium and depletion of the total body potassium content.

- No glucose gets into cells without insulin
- Fat breaks down to feed cells
- Ketones are created as by-product
- Ketones are acid
- Acidosis causes hyperkalemia and hyperventilation
- Kidneys excrete potassium

### Things You Will Be Asked on Rounds

- Bicarbonate, glucose, and potassium levels
- Low pH
- Whether at least 1–2 liters of IV saline has been given
- Next set of labs ordered
- ICU consult been called
- Whether it is known why patient is in DKA

Patients with diabetes don't just develop DKA without a reason. You must try to find that reason before you present to your team. You will be asked! If you do not identify the reason for DKA, you can't correct it. If you do not correct the reason for DKA, it will recur. The most common reasons for DKA are:

- Running out of or inability to take usual medications
- Infection (stress hormones inhibit insulin)
- Any major illness such as myocardial infarction, pancreatitis, or stroke
- New onset disease

### Round Saver

Know the insurance type. How does the patient pay for his medications?

DKA, by definition, presents with:

- Metabolic acidosis (low pH <7.2–7.3)
- Low serum bicarbonate
- Respiratory alkalosis ($pCO_2$ <35–40 mmHg) as compensation
- Anion gap elevation (>12 mEq/L)
- Hyperglycemia may exceed 700–800 mg/dL

Anion gap = $Na^+$ minus ($Cl^-$ and $HCO_3^-$)

DKA usually presents with:

- Ketones in blood and urine (presence in blood much more important)
- Not all ketones (e.g., beta-hydroxybutyrate) are measured
- Glucose in urine
- Low sodium from hyperglycemia (pseudohyponatremia); for each increase in glucose above normal of 100 mg/dL, there is a 1.6 drop in sodium
- Leukocytosis
- Elevated hemoglobin A1c (HbA1c)

**No other disease requires as frequent a repeat of testing as DKA.** Though the initial treatment of high volume of several liters of fluid and insulin is clear, it is not clear how much insulin is needed later or how long the person needs to stay in the ICU. For pH in DKA, a venous blood gas is equal to an arterial blood gas.

Do the following tests at least every 2–4 hours for the first 24 hours in the ICU:

- Serum bicarbonate
- Glucose
- Venous or arterial blood gas
  - Do not rely on $HCO_3^-$ levels in a blood gas; they are calculated, not directly measured
- Potassium level

**Round Saver**

When uncertain in DKA, repeat the glucose, $K^+$, and $HCO_3^-$ levels

For treatment, move patient to ICU until most of the acidosis resolves.

- Normal saline in high volumes: 1–2 liters per hour for the first 2–3 hours
- IV insulin: 0.05–0.1 units per kilogram per hour
- IV bicarbonate may be used when pH <7.0–7.1

Acidosis causes hyperkalemia, and hyperkalemia leads to increased urinary loss of potassium. Urinary loss of potassium thus decreases total body potassium level.

When acidosis resolves with treatment, hypokalemia will occur unless it is replaced.

If treated with several liters of fluid, insulin, and frequent monitoring, DKA will promptly resolve over 12–24 hours. You will feel very satisfied when you see:

- Serum bicarbonate rising >18–22 mEq/L
- pH rising >7.3
- Potassium level <4.5–5 mEq/L
- Glucose level <250 mg/dL

When this happens, you can do the following:

- Switch IV insulin off
- Start subcutaneous insulin
- Add potassium to IV fluids when it comes to <4.5 mEq/L
- Add glucose or dextrose to the IV fluids
- Transfer the patient to the floor

## Nonketotic Hyperosmolar Syndrome

When glucose levels are markedly elevated but there are no ketones and serum bicarbonate is normal, **nonketotic hyperosmolar syndrome** will result. Treatment is the same as DKA in terms of:

- High volume IV normal saline
  - Do not be afraid to use at least 1–2 liters/hr for several hours in a row
- Insulin

The difference is that there is a **normal anion gap**, **normal serum bicarbonate**, and **normal potassium level**.

## Inpatient Management of DM

With 10,000 new patients diagnosed per week in the United States because of increasing obesity, DM is one of the most common diseases you will see on your rotation. The most important part of management is whether the serum bicarbonate is normal. If so, the patient can be managed on the regular hospital floor.

- Do **not** stop all the usual outpatient medications on admission.
- Do **not** stop all the oral diabetic medications.
- Even if the patient is NPO, cut the insulin dose in half and cover with "finger-sticks" and a sliding scale of insulin. This is true even if the patient is going to the operating room.
- You **must** know the list of outpatient medications so you can continue them.
- You **must** know the starting and maximum doses of all diabetic medications the patient is using.
- You cannot know when to add or increase a medication if you do not know the dosing.
- Expect the glucose levels to be different in hospital than at home.
- If NPO, glucose will be lower than at home.
- If on IV fluids, glucose levels will be higher than at home.

**Round Saver**

Prior to rounds, always look up the doses of all your patients' meds.

### Lab Values for DM

Don't go to rounds without having looked up the labs on your patient. No one expects you to know all the plans for the future, but there is absolutely no excuse for not knowing the past history and current labs.

- Finger-stick values for last 48 hours
- Last serum glucose
- Last hemoglobin A1c as an outpatient (ask about it!)

- Know whether labs were ordered and drawn that morning
- Have medications been given in hospital? Not just "ordered," but confirmed as having been given?

## Other Considerations for DM

Depending on the other reasons for hospitalization and the glucose level, there may be no additional therapy needed. This is why it is absolutely essential to call the patient's primary care doctor.

A call to the primary doctor is essential because oral hypoglycemic agents can take weeks to adjust. Any medications you order will need to be adjusted by the outpatient doctor. Moreover, if you do not tell the patient's primary doctor what you ordered and why, he or she will only stop or alter the treatment. It frequently happens that a patient is admitted and the glucose control is poor. Your team will wonder, "Why wasn't more treatment given?" Only a call to the regular doctor can tell you:

- Was the patient previously administered the drug your team is contemplating?
- Has there been intolerance of this class before?
- Is there an extenuating circumstance such as loss or limitation of insurance or income?

| Commonly Used Oral Hypoglycemic Agents | | |
|---|---|---|
| **Drug Class** | **Doses in Milligrams** | **Contraindications** |
| Metformin | 500 bid start<br>2,500/day maximum | Renal insufficiency |
| Sulfonylurea | Glyburide: 2.5 to 20, 1x or 2x/day<br>Glimepiride: 2 to 4, 1x/day<br>Glipizide: 2.5 to 20, 1x or 2x/day | Hypoglycemia |
| Thiazolidinediones | Rosiglitazone: 2 to 8, 1x/day<br>Pioglitazone: 15 to 45, 1x/day | CHF |
| DPP-4 inhibitor | Sitagliptin: 25 to 100, 1x/day<br>Saxagliptin: 2.5 to 5, 1x/day<br>Linagliptin: 5, 1x/day | Pancreatitis |

DPP-4 = dipeptidyl peptidase 4

## Ambulatory Management of DM

Many patients with diabetes mellitus (DM) are asymptomatic and diagnosed when glucose is found to be elevated on routine testing. Look for an obese patient with polyuria, polydipsia, and polyphagia.

Screening is controversial. It is not entirely clear which patient groups should be screened. The clearest indication for screening is in those who are:

- Hypertensive
- Obese
- Age >45
- Have significant family history

Diagnostic criteria are as follows:

- Hemoglobin A1c >6.5%
- Fasting blood glucose >125 mg/dL on 2 measurements
- Single glucose level >200 mg/dL with symptoms
- Oral glucose tolerance test 2-hour postprandial >200 mg/dL

Treatment includes diet, exercise, and weight loss. Done together, these changes will prevent 25% of patients from ever needing medication.

- Start with metformin 500 mg bid.
    - Avoid with renal insufficiency because it may lead to metabolic or lactic acidosis.
- Sulfonylurea, thiazolidinedione, or DPP-4 inhibitor can be added.
- If 3 or 4 of the oral medications are not effective in controlling glucose to HgA1c <7%, switch to insulin or add insulin.
    - An alternative to insulin is an incretin-mimetic agent such as exenatide or liraglutide.

Incretin drugs are glucose-dependent insulinotropic peptide (GIP) and "glucagon-like" peptide (GLP). Both GIP and GLP will increase insulin from the pancreas and decrease glucagon. You can decrease the metabolism of incretins with DPP-4 inhibitors (sitagliptin, saxagliptin, or linagliptin) or you can replace them with exenatide or liraglutide.

Exenatide and liraglutide are longer-acting versions of the natural incretins (GLP). They increase insulin, grow the pancreas, decrease glucagon, and slow gastric motility. Exenatide is an injection.

## Long-Term Management of DM

In addition to glucose management, prevention of diabetic complications to the eye, feet, heart, brain, and kidney is the most important thing you can do with diabetes.

- **Blood pressure:** ACE inhibitor or angiotensin receptor blocker (ARB) to goal <130/80 mmHg
- **LDL:** statin to goal <100 mg/dL
- **Urine:** microalbumin screening annually
  - Use ACEI or ARB if present
  - "Micro" albumin is a level too low to be found on urinalysis (UA). Do UA first; if negative, send urine annually for microalbuminuria.
- **Eye:** Annual examination by ophthalmology for retinopathy with a dilated examination. Proliferative retinopathy is referred to ophthalmology for laser photocoagulation. Proliferative retinopathy is defined as neovascularization or vitreous hemorrhages
- **Foot exam:** Microfilament for detection of neuropathy of the feet

# THYROID DISORDERS

Although extremely common, there is no routine screening of the general population for thyroid disorders. Early detection does not alter much in an asymptomatic person.

## Hypothyroidism and Hyperthyroidism

With **hypothyroidism**, everything is slow. With **hyperthyroidism**, everything is fast.

As the first tests, do a thyroid stimulating hormone (TSH) and free T4 level. Thyroid antibodies are minimally altered and are generally "the most common wrong answer." Do not treat empirically; get diagnosis first.

| | Hypothyroid | Hyperthyroid |
|---|---|---|
| **Pulse** | Slow, bradycardia | Fast, tachycardia |
| **Weight** | Gain | Loss |
| **Bowel** | Constipation | Increased frequency |
| **Skin** | Dry | Sweaty |
| **Psychiatric** | Depression, dementia | Anxiety, nervousness |
| **Bone** | None | Osteoporosis |
| **Menstruation** | Menorrhagia | Oligomenorrhea |

## Diagnostic Testing

**Hypothyroidism:** Because almost all hypothyroidism is from primary gland failure, tests show **low free T4** and **elevated TSH**.

Antibody testing and low T3 levels add little to this. The reason is because most hypothyroidism is from simple gland "failure," which likely represents a "burnt out" Hashimoto's thyroiditis. These patients often never feel a hyperthyroid phase of the disease and just come to the clinic or the office with fatigue.

**Hyperthyroidism:** Tests show elevated T4 in hyperthyroidism of any type.

The other diagnostic test differences for thyroid disorders are:

| | Graves' Disease | Silent "Painless" Thyroiditis | Subacute Thyroiditis | Pituitary Adenoma | Synthroid (Thyroid Hormone) Abuse |
|---|---|---|---|---|---|
| **TSH** | Low | Low | Low | **High** | Low |
| **RAIU** | **High** | Low | Low | High | Low |
| **Key Features** | Eye & skin findings | Nontender | **Tenderness** | None | Involuted, nonpal-pable gland |
| **Anti-bodies** | TSI | | | | |

RAIU = radioactive iodine uptake; TSI = thyroid-stimulating immunoglobulin

Exophthalmos (proptosis) is seen only in **Graves' disease**.

## Treatment

**Hypothyroidism:** Replace the hormone (levothyroxine/Synthroid).

- Allow 6–8 weeks between dosing changes because it is slow.
- Use both TSH and free-T4 levels as follow-up for a response.
- Go slow with coronary disease; ischemia can be provoked if level is raised too fast.

For chronic treatment:

- Graves' disease: radioactive iodine ablates the gland
- Subacute thyroiditis: aspirin for pain
- Silent "painless" thyroiditis: resolves spontaneously
- Pituitary adenoma: transsphenoidal surgery

**Severe hyperthyroidism (thyroid storm):** Beta blockers are the fastest treatment. Propranolol is most often used but metoprolol is also acceptable. Beta blockers stop the action at the target organ.

- Beta blockers (propranolol, metoprolol)
- Propylthiouracil or methimazole (stops production and conversion of T4 to T3)
- Steroids (stop peripheral conversion)
- Iodinated contrast agents (stop uptake of iodine into gland); stop conversion

Surgery is done only in cases of pregnancy or where compression of the airway is present.

## Thyroid Nodules

Nodules are extremely common; as many as 5% of all women get thyroid nodules. If a nodule is found, do the following:

- Check the TSH and free T4.
- If hyperthyroid, treat the hyperthyroidism.
- If TSH and T4 are normal, biopsy the nodule.
    - Fine-needle aspiration is sufficient.
- If "follicular adenoma" is found, perform an excisional biopsy.

Nuclear thyroid scans are not helpful with thyroid nodules. They are not sensitive enough to exclude cancer.

Thyroid sonogram is used only to guide where to place the needle for a biopsy. Sonogram is not sufficient to exclude cancer.

Remember, needle the nodule. Nodules need needles!

# ADRENAL DISORDERS

## Hypercortisolism

The most challenging part of hypercortisolism is the diagnostic testing. You are far more likely to encounter drug-induced hypercortisolism from treatment than you are to find Cushing's syndrome from a pituitary or adrenal disorder.

On your Medicine rotation, laboratory testing is so pervasive and extensive that it is ridiculous to talk about 19th-century findings of just altered body habitus. The asymptomatic elevation in the white blood cell count is just as important a presentation as truncal obesity.

### Presentation

- Fat redistribution such as truncal and facial obesity ("moon face") with thin arms and legs
- Easy bruising and osteoporosis from protein breakdown for gluconeogenesis
- Menstrual abnormalities
- Acne from the overproduction of adrenal androgens
- Hypertension (cortisol increases sodium reabsorption and potentiates the effects of catecholamines on vasculature)
- Leukocytosis
- Hyperglycemia and hyperlipidemia
- Metabolic alkalosis (aldosterone excretes acid)
- Hypokalemia (aldosterone excretes potassium)
- Prednisone, dexamethasone, or methylprednisolone in the history

Hypercortisolism comes with an increased aldosterone effect as well.

## Diagnostic Testing

In endocrinology, never start with a scan. To confirm the presence of hypercortisolism, do a 24-hour urine cortisol and a 1-mg overnight dexamethasone suppression test. These tests are used to prove that there is hypercortisolism. A normal 1-mg overnight dexamethasone suppression test excludes hypercortisolism. If 24-hour cortisol is elevated, there is definitely hypercortisolism, though it won't tell you whether it is from:

- Pituitary adenoma
- Adrenal adenoma
- Ectopic production (e.g., carcinoid)

There are more false-positive test results from the 1-mg overnight dexamethasone suppression than for any other test. Anxiety, depression, alcoholism, and any other "stress in your head" has a physiologic manifestation that simulates adrenal hypersecretion. The 24-hour urine test encompasses cortisol levels during sleep as well. Therefore, if someone's anxiety is reduced, urine levels will go down during sleep. If the cause is an adenoma, however, there will still be hypersecretion even when asleep.

To determine the source of the hypercortisolism, do the following:

If the 24-hour urine cortisol is elevated, do an ACTH test:

- If ACTH is down, the source is adrenal (e.g., adrenal adenoma).
- If ACTH is up, the source is pituitary adenoma, of ectopic nature, or cancer.

If the ACTH level is elevated, do a high-dose dexamethasone test:

- If dexamethasone suppresses ACTH, the source is pituitary adenoma.
- If dexamethasone does not suppress ACTH, the source is of ectopic nature or cancer.

### Treatment

Remove whatever you find surgically. After doing the biochemical tests above, scan the area you identify as the source.

- Adrenal adenoma: laparoscopic adrenalectomy
- Pituitary adenoma: transsphenoidal pituitary removal (hypophysectomy)
- Ectopic focus in the lung or cancer: remove

## Hyperaldosteronism (Conn's Syndrome)

Hyperaldosteronism presents with:

- Hypertension
- Hypokalemia
- Metabolic alkalosis

Because water is absorbed with the sodium, the sodium level is normal. There is also a "sodium escape" into the urine. Although aldosterone increases sodium absorption and both potassium and hydrogen excretion, you should expect a normal serum sodium.

Lots of patients have hypertension. Be on the lookout for "I feel weak" and a decrease in muscle strength. These happen from low potassium levels. Hypokalemia impairs muscle contraction.

### Diagnostic Testing

Confirm with a low renin level combined with a high aldosterone level. Scan the adrenals with CT.

- Solitary adrenal adenoma: 85%
- Bilateral hyperplasia: 10–15%
- Cancer: 1%

### Treatment

- Laparoscopy (adenoma and cancer)
- Lifelong spironolactone or eplerenone to inhibit (bilateral hyperplasia)

## Hypoadrenalism (Addison's Disease)

Addison's disease is usually caused by autoimmune adrenal destruction. It presents with:

- Weakness, fatigue, and lack of energy
- Hyperpigmentation of skin from increased ACTH with primary adrenal failure
- Hypotension
- Hyperkalemia and metabolic acidosis

Test with cosyntropin stimulation. Measure the cortisol level before and after giving ACTH or cosyntropin. A normal response is a rise in cortisol. There is no rise in cortisol after injecting cosyntropin.

### Treatment

- Hydrocortisone, prednisone, and possibly fludrocortisone
- Fludrocortisone is the steroid with the highest mineralocorticoid or aldosterone-like effect.

## Pheochromocytoma

With pheochromocytoma, there are no distinct or unique physical findings. Look for:

- Episodic hypertension
- Flushing, headache, sweating, and tachycardia
- Failure of control with 3+ medications

### Diagnostic Testing

The best initial tests are 24-hour urine catecholamines and metanephrines (98% sensitive and specific). Also, plasma metanephrines should be done.

Confirm the location with an abdominal CT scan. If the scan can't find location but the metanephrine and catecholamine tests suggest it is indeed there, do an MIBG scan. An MIBG scan will detect occult pheochromocytoma not found on abdominal CT.

Treat with phenoxybenzamine and propranolol prior to surgical removal.

## Adrenal "Incidentaloma"

It is extremely common to find adrenal lesions on abdominal CT done for other reasons in those without symptoms referable to the adrenal. A lesion found on CT of the adrenals done for symptoms of pheochromocytoma, hypercortisolism, or hyperaldosteronism is NOT an "incidentaloma." The term *incidentaloma* specifically refers to a CT or MRI done for reasons other than adrenal lesion symptoms.

These lesions are found in 4% of the general population and in as many as 10% of older patients.

Benign lesions:

- Small (<4 cm)
- Round
- Smooth
- Low density

Malignant lesions:

- Large (>4 cm)
- Irregular
- High density

## Diagnostic Testing

Lesions suggestive of malignancy should undergo CT-guided needle biopsy. All benign-appearing lesions need tests to exclude subclinical endocrine functionality.

- Nonfunctional: 90%
- Cushing's: 6%
- Pheochromocytoma: 3%
- Aldosteronism: 1%

Do the 1-mg overnight dexamethasone suppression test and 24-hour urine metanephrine and catecholamine tests. For hypertensive patients, do a plasma aldosterone:renin ratio even if the serum potassium level is normal.

To treat, remove any malignant or endocrinologically functional lesion.

# Congenital Adrenal Hyperplasia

Congenital adrenal hyperplasia (CAH) is almost exclusively an ambulatory management issue. It is caused by enzymatic deficiencies in the adrenal gland which, when partial, may not present until adulthood. The overproduction of adrenal androgens such as DHEA or androstenedione will not be noticeable in men, but it will lead to clitoromegaly, deep voice, abnormal increase in hair, and masculinization in women.

| Enzyme Deficiency | Hypertension | Virilization |
| --- | --- | --- |
| **21**-hydroxylase | No | Yes |
| **11**-hydroxylase | Yes | Yes |
| **17**-hydroxylase | Yes | No |

About 95% of CAH is due to 21-OH deficiency.

### Diagnostic Testing

All 3 forms of CAH have high ACTH, low aldosterone, and low cortisol. 21-hydroxylase deficiency has a massive increase in 17-hydroxyprogesterone levels.

Treatment for all 3 forms of CAH is glucocorticoids, which provide feedback inhibition on ACTH.

## Hypercalcemia

The most common cause of hypercalcemia is hyperparathyroidism for outpatients and malignancy for inpatients. Other causes are:

- Vitamin D intoxication
- Sarcoidosis and granulomatous diseases
- Thiazide diuretics
- Vitamin A toxicity
- Lithium
- Hyperthyroidism

**Round Saver**

You must try to ascribe a clear cause to every lab abnormality you encounter.

Hypercalcemia, particularly from hyperparathyroidism, is often found on serum chemistry testing done for other reasons. Patients are asymptomatic. You will often find it on the routine chemistry testing done on patients being admitted to the hospital. When the calcium level comes up as elevated, you must quickly run through the list above in order to ascribe a clear cause.

The next step is to ask, "Is the patient symptomatic?" Symptomatic patients can never wait for a clear diagnosis to start treatment.

## Things You Will Be Asked on Rounds

- Kidney stones
- Blood in the urine
- Pain on the sides
- Difficulty with a bowel movement; frequency of bowel movements per day
- Belly pain
- Confusion at times or a look of sleepiness or disorientation
- History of bone fracture without trauma; spine or vertebral fracture
- Nephrogenic diabetes insipidus (NDI)
    - Frequent trips to the bathroom without having had a lot of water
    - Frequency of peeing throughout the night
- Muscle weakness; recent difficulty carrying bags home

Diabetes insipidus (DI) is a major cause of volume depletion.

Other manifestations of hypercalcemia are:

- Renal tubular acidosis (look for low serum bicarbonate with normal anion gap)
- Chloride level will be high
- Ulcers: calcium stimulates release of gastrin
- Pancreatitis

## How NOT to Kill Your Patient

- Give massive amounts of IV fluids for DI
- Recheck sodium and calcium levels

## Diagnostic Testing

Know these tests before rounds and presentations:

- BUN and creatinine: hypercalcemia is associated with renal toxicity
- EKG: hypercalcemia gives short QT while hypocalcemia gives long QT
- Sodium level: hypercalcemia causes nephrogenic diabetes insipidus (DI)
- Urinalysis
- Phosphate level: will be down in hyperparathyroidism

The use of lithium, vitamin D, vitamin A, and thiazide diuretics should be obvious, if you ask about them. If these agents are not being used and there is no malignancy, the next test is a parathyroid hormone (PTH) level. High calcium along with high PTH means primary hyperparathyroidism.

You do not have to go on a search for cancer if it is not obvious from the history beyond the screening mammography, colonoscopy, and Pap smear, which everyone should have. The hypercalcemia of malignancy is rare from small, localized, or solitary lesions. It is usually from metastatic disease that should be clear once you ask.

If the diagnosis is not clear after the history and parathyroid hormone level are done, obtain a 24-hour urine for calcium in outpatients to look for familial hypocalciuric hypercalcemia.

For severe calcium disorders, get an EKG.

## Treatment

For **symptomatic**, **acute hypercalcemia**, treat with the following:

- Fluids at high volume: normal saline 200–500 mL/hr for several hours
- Bisphosphonates (need 1–2 days to work)

- Calcitonin if level is still high after hydration while waiting for bisphosphonates to work
- Glucocorticoids (only for sarcoidosis and granulomatous diseases)
- Bisphosphonates
  - Zoledronic acid 4 mg over 15 minutes
  - Pamidronate 60–90 mg

Loop diuretics are not a good idea unless there is CHF or renal insufficiency and the likelihood of fluid overload.

For **hyperparathyroidism**, treat with the following:

- Surgical removal is the only treatment. Solitary adenoma causes 80% of cases. Surgery is indicated for:
  - All symptomatic patients (e.g., confusion, abdominal pain)
  - Nephrogenic diabetes insipidus
  - Renal stones or decreased renal function
  - Osteoporosis and bone lesions
  - Young patients (age <50) with calcium levels >1 point above normal
- Four-gland hyperplasia requires removal of all 4 glands and lifelong calcium and vitamin D replacement

## Hypocalcemia

Asymptomatic hypocalcemia is common. First check the albumin level. A low albumin level will lower the total calcium level. Free calcium will be normal.

> **Round Saver**
>
> Calcium is down 0.8 for every 1.0 point below normal of albumin.

Low free calcium presents with neuromuscular hyperexcitability, such as:

- Seizures and psychiatric manifestations

- Cardiac arrhythmia from prolonged QT: get an EKG
- Facial nerve tetany ("Chvostek's sign"): tap on the face by the ear
- Perioral numbness and tingling: from alkalosis of hyperventilation in a panic attack

## Etiology

- Renal failure: 1,25-dihydroxy vitamin D deficiency
- Vitamin D deficiency (nutritional or resistance)
- Hypomagnesemia: failure of release of PTH
- Hypoparathyroidism: from surgery, neck radiation, autoimmune destruction
- Drug induced: phenytoin (damages vitamin D), foscarnet, cinacalcet inhibits PTH release

Phosphate is up when low calcium is caused by renal failure.

Treatment for acute symptomatic hypocalcemia is IV calcium gluconate or calcium chloride. There is no maximum on IV replacement rate. For chronic disease, give oral calcium, often with vitamin D.

# PITUITARY DISORDERS

The most common presentation of a pituitary lesion is galactorrhea, menstrual, or erectile dysfunction from hyperprolactinemia. The functional manifestations of hyperprolactinemia or acromegaly are more common than the mass effect of the lesion on the optic chiasm. Since **micro**adenomas are more common than **macro**adenomas, headache and visual disturbance such as bitemporal hemianopsia are rare.

## Hyperprolactinemia

Lesions present with:

- Menstrual irregularity or amenorrhea
- Galactorrhea in women
- Erectile dysfunction
- Infertility from inhibition of GnRH

### Diagnostic Testing

In endocrinology, never start with a scan. If there is evidence of hyperprolactinemia, then:

- Exclude pregnancy
- Measure prolactin level
- Look for causes of hyperprolactinemia other than a pituitary lesion
  - Pregnancy
  - Hypothyroidism: thyrotropin-releasing hormone (TRH) from the hypothalamus stimulates prolactin when at pathologically high levels
  - Medications: phenothiazine psychiatric medications inhibit dopamine, SSRIs, metoclopramide, opiates, verapamil, cimetidine
  - Chest wall injury or excess stimulation, zoster of the chest
  - Estrogen (this is the substance that normally raises prolactin during pregnancy)
  - Renal failure

When prolactin level is high, and pregnancy and other causes of hyperprolactinemia have been excluded, do an MRI of the pituitary.

Do not start with an MRI of the pituitary. Around 10% of patients will have a pituitary lesion. Confirm biochemically first, then do an MRI.

### Treatment

- Dopamine-agonist medications:
  - Cabergoline
  - Bromocriptine
- Transsphenoidal surgery to remove the lesion
- Radiation only as a last resort

## Acromegaly

Growth hormone increases insulin-like growth factor (IGF). IGF grows proteins in numerous sites of the body. In addition to enlargement of the hat, ring, and shoe size from head, hand, and foot size, other abnormalities of acromegaly are:

- Cardiomyopathy
- Increased sweating: sweat glands enlarge
- Colonic polyps, including increased risk of colon cancer
- Nerve entrapment such as carpal tunnel from surrounding tissue pressing on the nerves
- Joint pain: bones and joints grow out of alignment
- Obstructive sleep apnea

Growth hormone has anti-insulin effects, which lead to coronary artery disease. The anti-insulin effects also lead to:

- Hyperglycemia
- Hyperlipidemia

### Diagnostic Testing

The best initial test is IGF level (long half-life). Growth hormone has a short half-life and is maximal in the middle of the night.

The best **confirmatory** test is glucose suppression. The normal response is a suppression of growth hormone by glucose. It fails to suppress with acromegaly.

Never start with a brain MRI scan, as 10% of patients have nonfunctional pituitary lesions.

### Treatment

- Transsphenoidal surgery to remove the pituitary gland
- Pegvisomant (growth hormone receptor antagonist), octreotide (somatostatin), or a dopamine agonist (e.g., cabergoline)

## Panhypopituitarism

Any damage to the pituitary from an infarction, infection, or surrounding mass effect from a tumor can damage the production and release of anterior pituitary hormones. The pituitary is a small, delicate organ that is easily compressed.

Patients with panhypopituitarism will present with adrenal insufficiency or hypothyroidism as previously described. The key issue is how to know that the etiology is specifically in the pituitary, though this changes little in management approach and need to replace glucocorticoids or thyroxine (T4).

## Diagnostic Testing

- ACTH, cortisol, TSH, T4, and IGF levels
  - Normal levels will exclude pituitary insufficiency. Provocative testing is done if the other hormone levels are equivocal.
- Arginine stimulation testing
  - With arginine, a normal response is an increase in growth hormone release.
- Metyrapone
  - This will inhibit 11-hydroxylase and reduce the cortisol level. A normal response is an increase in ACTH level. Cortisol is feedback on the pituitary. Metyrapone shuts off the cortisol and thus a normal response is for ACTH level to rise.

## Empty Sella Syndrome

Look for obese women with a headache. Empty sella syndrome is often found on CT or MRI of the brain done for other reasons. This is an anatomic variant that needs no treatment.

## Kallmann Syndrome

- Hypogonadotropin
- Low FSH and LH levels
- Anosmia

Treat with sex hormone replacement.

## Diabetes Insipidus

Diabetes insipidus (DI) is caused by an insufficient amount or action of antidiuretic hormone (ADH).

**Central DI:** insufficient ADH production from any cause of CNS damage

- Trauma
- Tumors
- Hypoxia
- Infection

**Nephrogenic diabetes insipidus (NDI)**

- Damage to the kidney
- Chronic pyelonephritis
- Sickle cell disease
- Hypercalcemia
- Hypokalemia
- Lithium

# Gastroenterology 3

## Gastrointestinal Bleeding

The most important feature of GI bleed is **severity**, not **etiology**. If the bleed is severe, first resuscitate with fluids and blood. The cause is important, but not as important as the severity.

Determine the severity of the bleed:

**SBP <90 mmHg = extremely severe bleeding**

| Hemodynamic Finding | Approximate Volume Loss |
|---|---|
| Blood donation | 10% |
| Orthostasis | 15–20% |
| Pulse >100/min | 30% |
| SBP <100 mmHg | 30% |

### How NOT to Kill Your Patient

- Make sure IV fluids have been started.
- What is the blood pressure? If systolic BP (SBP) <90–95 mmHg, **stop reading this book** and get your resident or attending to order 500 mL of normal saline (NS) **immediately**.
- Make sure CBC has been sent, checked, and repeated.
- If platelets <30,000–50,000 $mm^3$ with severe bleeding, ask about immediate platelet transfusion
- Prothrombin time (PT) or INR: No amount of endoscopy stops bleeding if there is a coagulation defect. If PT or INR is increased, give FFP.
- Has a proton pump inhibitor (PPI) been started? (all upper GI bleeds)
- There is no such thing as "too much fluid" if SBP <90 mmHg.
- Make sure a type and cross for packed red blood cell (PRBC) transfusion has been sent.

## Orthostatic Hypotension

"Orthostatic" means that at rest while lying flat, the patient's blood pressure and pulse are normal, and when sitting or standing up, blood pressure drops and pulse goes up. Orthostatic hypotension is an indispensible evaluation of severity. Many patients will be admitted in whom you are not sure if the bleeding is severe because blood pressure and pulse at rest are normal. Orthostatic evaluation will identify who has a minor bleed and who has a severe one.

It takes 6–12 hours to follow CBCs over time to see if there is a drop in hematocrit consistent with severe bleeding. If there is no orthostasis on initial evaluation, you can feel confident the bleeding is not severe. Check for orthostasis right away before a lot of fluids are given.

Do not be surprised if you, the less experienced medical student, are the FIRST person to think of doing orthostasis. Attendings and nurses often forget to check orthostatics. **Orthostasis** is a drop in blood pressure or rise in pulse upon standing or sitting.

Systolic blood pressure **decrease** >20 mmHg or pulse **increase** >10/min

For severe bleeding, give:

- Fluids
- Blood
- Platelets
- Plasma

## Esophageal Varices

- Octreotide needs to be added immediately.
- Banding is indispensible. (Make sure GI service has been called, as banding can only be done with endoscopy.)
  - Do sclerotherapy only if banding cannot be done.
- Beta blockers (propranolol and nadolol) do nothing for acute variceal bleeding.

One CBC cannot determine the severity of bleeding. To repeat, one CBC cannot determine the severity of bleeding!

> **Round Saver**
>
> Hematocrit drops only 2–3 points with hydration.

If bleeding is severe, make sure the GI service has been called. Make sure to indicate if the bleeding is severe. You will be asked to provide CBC, PT/INR, blood pressure, and response to fluids.

- EKG: Severe anemia and GI bleeding kills you via myocardial ischemia. Lightheadedness does not kill you.
- Anyone with symptomatic anemia needs a transfusion. Now!
- Symptoms of anemia are lightheadedness, dyspnea, fatigue, and chest pain.

Fluid replacement is more important than scoping.

### Things You Will Be Asked on Rounds

In evaluating GI bleed, the first step is to establish the severity. Ask the following questions WHILE you are checking for orthostasis:

- Time when bleeding started
- Is stool red or black?
- Are you vomiting bright red blood or dark "coffee grounds"?
- Number of bowel movements or episodes of vomiting with blood or black stool
- Lightheadedness, shortness of breath, chest pain
- History of heart disease
- Previous scope through the mouth or rectum
- Antacid use

## Etiology

### Round Saver

Check for orthostasis **yourself**.

**Lower GI bleed** can stem from any of the following:

- Diverticulosis
- Angiodysplasia or "arteriovenous malformation" (AVM)
- Polyps
- Cancer

Lower bleed gives bright red blood on bowel movement. Upper GI bleed can be red if it is extremely severe and fast in about 10% of cases.

**Hemorrhoid bleed** can easily be mistaken for serious GI bleed. A small amount of red blood into the toilet bowel makes the water look red and exaggerates the severity of the blood loss. Hemorrhoid bleed has the following features:

- No change in hematocrit with repeated testing
- Hemorrhoids found on rectal exam
- Normal BP and pulse
- Absence of orthostatic change in blood pressure or pulse

Guaiac-positive, brown stool is not severe.

**Upper GI bleed** can stem from any of the following:

- Ulcer disease: both duodenal and gastric ulcers
- Gastritis
- Esophagitis
- Duodenitis
- Varices
- Cancer

> **Round Saver**
> Always ask "What will you do differently based on *that* test?"

Ulcer disease is the most common cause of upper GI bleed, though varices are the most dangerous. Both esophageal and gastric varices occur from portal hypertension. There is no way to be sure which of these is the precise cause without endoscopy.

Initial management of all of these conditions is identical, based on severity with IV fluids, frequent checking of CBC, and correction of coagulopathy. Continue to repeat CBC until it stops changing.

- Proton-pump inhibitors (PPIs) for all upper GI bleeds
- Epinephrine injection or electrocautery for ulcers with active bleeding

Nasogastric tube adds nothing to UGI bleeding management.

With **variceal bleed** you do not need to wait for endoscopy to confirm varices in order to start octreotide. Octreotide decreases portal pressure and has no major adverse effects.

- Band varices that bleed; gastric varices are hard to "grab" to band.
- Propranolol or nadolol is used **only to prevent the next bleed.**

Persistent bleeds, despite banding and octreotide, need transjugular intrahepatic portosystemic shunt (TIPS). TIPS involves a catheter down the jugular vein to create a small "shunt" between the portal and hepatic veins. This replaces the need for surgical shunting.

A Blakemore tube is a balloon placed into the esophagus and stomach to "tamponade," or "compress," the vessels. This is a temporary method of slowing bleeding in those who need to be kept alive for a few hours until TIPS can be done.

## Minor GI Bleed

Many patients in the clinic or office have minor GI bleeding characterized by guaiac (heme) positive stool. There is often a microcytic anemia as well. Those with epigastric discomfort should be scoped from above first. If there are no localizing symptoms, these patients need:

1. Colonoscopy
2. Upper endoscopy
3. Rarely, pill endoscopy, in those in whom endoscopy does not show the cause

Minor bleeding =

- Normal BP/pulse
- No orthostasis
- No recent change in hematocrit

## Epigastric Pain

Epigastric pain is benign in the majority of patients. The epigastric area is at the top of the abdomen just below the xiphoid process. It is sometimes called "dyspepsia." Pathology will never be found in 50–90% of outpatients; however, patients admitted for epigastric pain are markedly skewed toward more serious pathology. With the exception of pancreatitis, all of these forms of pain do not have tenderness on examination.

> **Round Saver**
>
> Your job is to find serious pathology by asking questions.

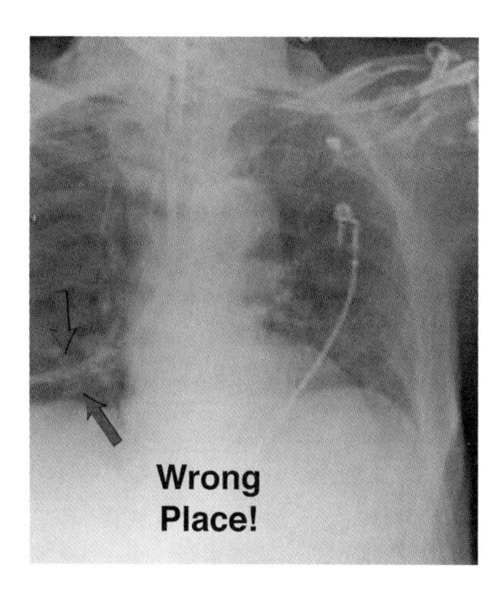


**Tube is misplaced in right lung. This is why x-ray is so important before tube feeding is started, and why routine NG tube in GI bleed is a bad idea.**

## Etiology

The most common cause of epigastric pain in the general population is "nonulcer dyspepsia" (NUD). NUD is pain without pathology. It is like tension headache of your guts. The inpatients on your Ward rotation will more likely have:

- Ulcer disease
- Pancreatitis
- Gastroesophageal reflux disease (GERD)
- Esophagitis/duodenitis/gastritis
- Cancer

To distinguish benign from dangerous disease, always ask about **duration, intensity, time of onset, and aggravating and relieving factors** for all pain syndromes. Specifically for epigastric pain, also ask:

- "Have you been **losing weight**?"
- "Have you actually weighed yourself? What is the exact amount you lost?"
- "How much did you weigh 6 months ago?"
- "Is it difficult for you to swallow? Does **food get "stuck"** when you eat?"
- "Do you have **pain when you swallow**?"
- "Are you nauseated? Do you actually vomit? How often?"
- "Do you have **blood in your stool** or when you vomit?"
- "Does the pain go away with antacids?"

**Round Saver** 

Find "alarm" symptoms!

- Weight loss
- Dysphagia
- Odynophagia
- Bleeding

## Diagnostic Testing

Esophagogastroduodenoscopy (EGD), the proper term for upper endoscopy, is essential in anyone with alarm symptoms. Your primary task is to identify those who need EGD. For patients without alarm symptoms, EGD is performed if age >45–55 or if symptoms persist or worsen despite the use of PPIs.

- Most accurate test of the stomach
- Allows banding of varices and cautery of visible vessels in an ulcer
- Needed for stomach biopsy to exclude cancer in gastric ulcer
- You cannot distinguish duodenal from gastric ulcer without endoscopy.

EGD is the **only way to exclude cancer.**

EGD is far more accurate than barium studies of the stomach. Because you cannot biopsy or perform therapeutic procedures with a barium study, this modality is rarely, if ever, used anymore. Ultimately, you can test and treat for *Helicobacter* without endoscopy but because 4% of gastric ulcer is associated with cancer, you are scoping to exclude the possibility of cancer.

***Helicobacter pylori* testing** is best done on biopsy.

- Important to drive treatment with PPI, clarithromycin, and amoxicillin
- *Helicobacter* stool antigen or breath testing is not as good as biopsy.
- Stool antigen and breath test **can differentiate** between old vs. current infection.
- **Serology is clinically useless.**
- Has no treatment benefit in GERD

Treat *H. pylori* only in those with ulcers or gastritis. Ulcers will recur if *H. pylori* is not eradicated.

## Stress Ulcer Prophylaxis

The *only* clear indications for stress ulcer prophylaxis are:

- Mechanical ventilation/Intubation
- Head trauma
- Burns
- Coagulopathy

You will see many, many patients placed on stress ulcer prophylaxis unnecessarily. NSAIDs and steroids are NOT indications for stress ulcer prophylaxis.

Although PPIs are generally benign, there is a slight risk of:

- *Clostridium difficile* colitis
- Osteoporosis from interference with calcium absorption
- Pneumonia: gastric acid protects against gastric colonization with bacteria

**Round Saver** 

Your duty to your patient is more important than always agreeing with your attending. Question every unnecessary test and treatment you see.

# Zollinger-Ellison Syndrome (ZES)

ZES is caused by **elevated gastric acid** and **elevated serum gastrin**. Look for ZES and get a gastrin level only if you see the following:

- Large ulcers (>1 cm)
- Recurrence after eradication of *H. pylori*
- Distal location near the far end of the duodenum near the ligament of Treitz
- Multiple ulcers

Diarrhea is frequent in ZES from the acid inactivation of lipase.

### Diagnostic Testing

- Serum gastrin level while patient is off PPIs and all forms of antacid
- Increased gastrin and gastric acid levels

Equivocal gastrin levels are confirmed with secretin testing. The normal response is a decrease in gastrin. In ZES, gastrin level stays high after giving secretin. Confirm that ZES is local and resectable by excluding metastases with endoscopic ultrasound and nuclear somatostatin receptor scan.

Local disease should be surgically removed. Use lifelong PPIs for metastatic or unresectable disease.

## Diabetic Gastroparesis

Long-standing diabetes damages nerves. Patients with this condition cannot feel the "stretch" of the bowel that is the main stimulant to GI motility. You will recognize it by:

- Bloating
- Nausea
- Constipation
- Abdominal discomfort

Manage diabetic gastroparesis by looking at the response to treatment with:

- Metoclopramide
- Erythromycin

A nuclear gastric emptying study can be used in those in whom the diagnosis is equivocal. Patients eat barium-soaked bread and are monitored for the time it takes for it to leave the stomach.

## Gastroesophageal Reflux Disease (GERD)

GERD develops because of an abnormally relaxed lower esophageal sphincter. Acid comes up out of the stomach and hits the back of the throat and vocal cords. GERD causes 25% of chronic cough.

### Things You Will Be Asked on Rounds

- "Does the pain/discomfort in your belly go anywhere? (like your chest?)"
- "Do you have 'heartburn'? Do you have pain in your chest?"
- "Do you have a bad taste in your mouth?"
- "Does it taste like metal? Like you have pennies in your mouth?"
- "Is your throat sore?"
- "Do you feel your voice is hoarse?"
- "Do you cough, especially at night?"

### Diagnostic Testing

GERD is rare in that the test generally is the response to treatment with PPIs. Because 95% of those with GERD should respond within a day to treatment with PPIs, only specific testing is performed in those with persistent symptoms.

- Start a PPI (they are all equal in efficacy).
- Ask later the same day if symptoms have improved.
- If symptoms persist, ask your resident/attending about performing EGD or 24-hour pH to look for another diagnosis.

**Round Saver**

*Helicobacter* does NOT cause GERD.

Surgical correction such as Nissen fundoplication is done for the small percentage (<5%) of patients not controlled with PPIs.

## Barrett's Esophagus

Barrett's esophagus can develop from long-standing GERD (usually >5 years). It is not always clear when to scope to screen GERD patients for Barrett's.

- Diagnosed by EGD: it can be seen and biopsy confirms.
- 0.5% patients a year develop adenocarcinoma.
- Biopsy is only way to confirm.

Treat with PPIs and repeat EGD every 2–3 years for early detection of cancer.

### Esophageal Dysplasia from Barrett's Esophagus

- Low-grade dysplasia: PPI and re-scope/re-biopsy every 6 months
- High-grade dysplasia: PPI and either endomucosal resection with endoscope or do distal esophagectomy
  - High-grade dysplasia must be physically removed before it becomes invasive cancer. Mucosal "shaves" with EGD are effective.

# Pancreatitis

Look for severe epigastric pain and **epigastric tenderness**. Pancreatitis can be incapacitating and worsens over hours to days.

- Gallstone disease is increasing because of obesity.
- Elevated amylase and lipase

Pancreatitis has tenderness on palpation.

### Things You Will Be Asked on Rounds

- Where the pain radiates
- Whether it goes **straight through to the back**
- Nausea and vomiting (if so, how many times, and is there blood?)
- Quantity of **alcohol** patient drinks
- History of **gallstones**

## Diagnostic Testing

Look for an increased amylase and lipase. Lipase is more specific, but generally both are done. Unfortunately residents and attending can torture you with learning the obsolete Ranson's Criteria, such as elevated WBC, low calcium, age >55, high AST, and high LDH. Ranson was a surgeon working before there were CT scans; these were the criteria he used to determine the need for surgical debridement.

- No test determines severity in first 48 hours.
- Although CT is most sensitive for confirming diagnosis, it is often unnecessary for that purpose.
- CT and US show the cause of pancreatitis such as stone or obstruction.
- Scanning is used to determine if stone removal is needed.
- MRCP (magnetic resonance cholangiopancreatography) is the diagnostic method that best visualizes ductal structure of the pancreas and biliary system.
- ERCP is the therapeutic method to remove stones and dilate strictures.

MRCP finds the obstruction while ERCP fixes it.

### Treatment

There is no medication that increases the speed of resolution of pancreatitis. Physicians provide "rest" of the pancreas and give a lot of fluid. Pancreatic inflammation releases a lot of mediators, which cause "leak" of capillaries. The main cause of death in acute pancreatitis is inadequate fluid replacement. Do not be afraid to give 150–250 mL per hour for the first day.

1. NPO (nil per os) or nothing to eat, IV fluids in large volumes, analgesics
2. Proton pump inhibitors are frequently used, though it is not clear they help
3. CT with >30% necrosis needs imipenem or meropenem and CT-guided biopsy.
4. Infected necrotic pancreatitis is rare but needs surgical debridement.

## Infectious Diarrhea

You never know the etiology of the diarrhea when the patient is admitted to the hospital. What matters is that you understand the severity of diarrhea, and especially, who needs antibiotics and IV fluids.

> **Round Saver**
> Blood in stool is the key to etiology.

To understand the severity of diarrhea:

**Severe = volume-depleted** and **febrile**

Refer to the GI bleeding section to precisely define "volume-depleted."

- Is SBP <90–100 mmHg? Is pulse >100/min?
- Check for orthostasis: increase in pulse >10 or drop in SBP >20 mmHg on rising
- Is there fever? (oral temperature >100.3°F)
- Is there blood in stool?
- Is there abdominal pain or tenderness on examination?

### Things You Will Be Asked on Rounds

- Duration of symptoms
- Frequency of bowel movements
- Blood in the stool
- Fever; has temperature been taken, or do you just feel warm?
- Lightheadedness
- Others that live with you who have the same problem/diarrhea
    - Did you eat at the same place? eat the same food?

## Diagnostic Testing

A precise microbiologic diagnosis is rarely confirmed, and decisions about treatment must be made before you have any test results back. Blood is only present with invasive pathogens such as *Campylobacter, Salmonella, Shigella, Yersinia,* or *Vibrio*. Blood may be present, however, only in microscopic or "occult" amounts in brown stool, but it gives the same information: invasive pathogens.

Fecal leukocytes (WBCs) have the same significance as blood, meaning an invasive pathogen is present. The only way to distinguish between these invasive pathogens is with stool culture.

If blood is not visible, do the following general tests in all patients:

- Occult blood (guaiac)
- Fecal leukocytes (methylene blue stain)
- Culture
- Ova and parasite exam

| History | Organism | Test |
| --- | --- | --- |
| AIDS <100 $CD_4$ cells | *Cryptosporidium* | Modified acid fast stain |
| Camper, hiker | *Giardia* | ELISA stool antigen, ova & parasite |
| Antibiotic use | *C. difficile* | Stool toxin assay |
| Hemolysis, low platelets, elevated BUN & creatinine | *E. coli* 0157:H7 | Sorbitol MacConkey agar |
| Flushing, wheezing immediately after fish eating | Scombroid | Stool culture |

## Treatment

The majority of infectious diarrhea cases are self-limited and benign; they require no antibiotic treatment. There is a much higher incidence of ciprofloxacin (fluoroquinolone) treatment in those admitted to hospital because that is the reason they have been admitted. Antimotility agents such as diphenoxylate (Lomotil) or loperamide (Imodium) can be used if there is no blood and no fever.

**Round Saver**

*E. coli* 0157:H7 does not grow on routine media!

Antibiotics are indicated in those with severe diarrhea. "Severe" is defined as a combination of the following:

- Fever
- Blood in stool
- Hypotension/tachycardia
- Abdominal pain or tenderness

**Round Saver**

Initial treatment is based on severity, not etiology.

### Pathogen-Specific Treatment

| Organism | Treatment |
|---|---|
| *C. difficile* | • Metronidazole first; vancomycin only if that fails<br>• Recurrences are treated with repeat course of metronidazole<br>• Very severe cases get both drugs |
| *Giardia* | Metronidazole, tinidazole |
| *Cryptosporidia* | Nitazoxanide |
| *Campylobacter* | Azithromycin or erythromycin if confirmed as *Campylobacter* |
| *E.coli* 0157:H7 | Avoid antibiotics |
| Scombroid | Diphenhydramine (antihistamine) |
| Viral, *Staph, Bacillus cereus* | • Supportive therapy with fluids<br>• Antibiotics do not help |

**Severe *C. difficile* is defined as:**

- Fever
- WBC >15,000–20,000/mm$^3$
- Creatinine >1.5 mg%
- >10 movements a day

## MALABSORPTIVE DISEASES

Fat malabsorption or steatorrhea is associated with weight loss and malabsorption of vitamin ADEK, which are the fat-soluble vitamins. Because of this, celiac disease, Whipple's disease, tropical sprue, and chronic pancreatitis have significant overlap in presentation. All of them present with:

- Weight loss
- Stool described as "oily, greasy, floating, and especially foul-smelling"
- Ask, "Do you bruise easily?" (vitamin K malabsorption)

- Look for bone disease such as osteoporosis (vitamin D malabsorption)
- Vitamin $B_{12}$ malabsorption leads to macrocytic/megaloblastic anemia
- Low calcium levels
- Stool: Sudan black stain positive (fecal fat test)

Fat malabsorption is accompanied by oily, greasy stool; weight loss; low $Ca^{++}$ and low $B_{12}$; and high PT.

## Celiac Disease

Celiac disease is also known as gluten-sensitive enteropathy. In addition to the weight loss and other signs of fat malabsorption described above, look for:

- Iron deficiency anemia (very common)
  - Celiac damages the duodenum
- Dermatitis herpetiformis: herpes-like lesions (not common)
- Small bowel lymphoma

Celiac disease has a strong association with diabetes. Eliminate gluten from the diet.

### Diagnostic Testing

Do serology tests first!

- Anti-tissue transglutaminase antibodies and anti-endomysial antibodies
- Anti-gliadin antibodies are imprecise
- Bowel biopsy (most accurate)
  - Look for flattened villi
  - Exclude bowel wall lymphoma

## Whipple's Disease

- Eye, joint, and neurologic manifestations
- Biopsy of bowel with PAS-positive organisms
- PCR or stool for *Tropheryma whippelii*
- Antibiotics for 6–12 months: ceftriaxone, doxycycline, TMP/SMX

## Chronic Pancreatitis

Ask about repeated episodes of pancreatitis over a period of years. In addition, chronic pancreatitis can have debilitating abdominal pain. Patients present with fat malabsorption from loss of lipase production. $B_{12}$ malabsorption occurs because pancreatic enzymes are needed to detach $B_{12}$ from R-protein to bind it to intrinsic factor.

### Diagnostic Testing

Calcification is present on abdominal x-ray in 50–60% and CT scan in 80–90%.

- Amylase and lipase levels are not elevated. The pancreas is "burnt out" and destroyed so there is no amylase or lipase left to release.
- Secretin stimulation testing is the most accurate test. IV secretin is given. The normal response is a massive release of pancreatic enzymes into the duodenum. In chronic pancreatitis, the pancreas is burnt out and there is no release of bicarbonate-rich fluid into the duodenum.

**Round Saver**

Expect normal amylase and lipase in chronic pancreatitis.

### Treatment

- Replace pancreatic enzymes orally.
- Lipase, trypsin, and amylase are easy to replace by pill.
- Pain managed with celiac ganglion block by injection via endoscopic ultrasound.

## Lactose Intolerance

Although lactose intolerance is extremely common, patients are never admitted to the hospital. Symptoms are diarrhea and gas. Lactose intolerance can be recognized by the following:

- No fever or blood in stool
- No weight loss
- No systemic manifestations
- Rapid resolution 1 day after stopping milk products (except yogurt)

Treatment is avoidance of milk products (including ice cream) or use of lactase replacement.

## Carcinoid Syndrome

Heart becomes fibrotic because of chronic neurotransmitter exposure.

- Episodic, chronic diarrhea
- Flushing, wheezing, and rarely right-sided cardiac fibrosis
- Telangiectasia from chronic flushing
- Metastatic lesions to liver are almost always present
- Urinary 5-HIAA level

Treatment is octreotide or lanreotide.

## Irritable Bowel Syndrome (IBS)

Patients with IBS are rarely admitted to the hospital, but many patients do seek help at the clinic. Nonspecific abdominal pain is extremely common. Your job is to make sure there is no serious pathology.

Diagnosis of IBS can only be made after testing is done. IBS is an abdominal pain syndrome with normal EGD, colonoscopy, and abdominal CT.

Look for abdominal pain with:

- Diarrhea or constipation, or diarrhea alternating with constipation
- Symptoms that are less severe at night
- Pain relieved by a bowel movement
- No weight loss
- No blood, mucous, or fever

### Treatment

IBS is extremely frustrating for the patient and the caregivers to treat. There is no single effective therapy, and you may notice staff being avoidant of these patients because they are in pain and there is no sure way to make it better. Start with the following:

- Fiber and bulking agents: Metamucil, psyllium husks, bran
- Anti-spasmodic agents: hyoscyamine or dicyclomine
- Tricyclic antidepressants

**Round Saver**

IBS is your chance to shine! With IBS patients, it is often only the students who have enough time and patience to stop and talk.

## Inflammatory Bowel Disease (IBD)

Ulcerative colitis (UC) and Crohn's disease (CD) collectively are called inflammatory bowel disease (IBD). Both are idiopathic disorders presenting with:

- Abdominal pain and diarrhea
- Blood and mucous in stool
- CD can have fever and palpable abdominal masses

Critical facts about IBD:

- Acute exacerbation means >10–20 bowel movements a day often with blood.
- Use steroids for acute episodes.
- Mesalamine is for long-term control.
- Fistulae of all kinds need TNF drugs such as infliximab.
- Screen for colon cancer after 10 years of colon involvement.

**Both UC and CD** can have:

- Joint pain
- Erythema nodosum/pyoderma gangrenosum
- Uveitis/episcleritis
- Sclerosing cholangitis (more common in UC)

**Round Saver**

Pyoderma and sclerosing cholangitis don't improve with disease control.

The following manifestations are **specific to CD:**

- Fistulae (from transmural granulomas): They can come through the skin or connect between loops of bowel or into the bladder.
- Perianal disease
- Oral, esophageal, and small bowel disease

## Diagnostic Testing

- Lower or upper endoscopy is first, depending on the symptoms.
- Small bowel series is sometimes needed for CD.

## Treatment

IBD exacerbation is like asthma. Use steroids in acute cases to calm it down.

- Steroids (for acute, severe exacerbations)
- Mesalamine (5-ASA) derivatives (for chronic control)
  - Asacol: for colonic involvement; used more with UC
  - Pentasa: works through entire bowel; used more with CD
  - Rowasa: rectal ASA; used only for those with limited distal/rectal disease
- Azathioprine/6-mercaptopurine (to wean patients off steroids and for chronic control)
- Anti-TNF medications such as infliximab, etanercept, adalimumab (for fistulae in CD)
- Ciprofloxacin and metronidazole (for perianal CD)
  - Besides being antibiotics, these medications have a primary anti-inflammatory effect.

### Screening for Colon Cancer with IBD

Both UC and CD cause colon cancer. Risk is based on the duration of involvement of the colon.

- CD with 10 years of colon involvement has the same risk as UC for 10 years.
- Whether the patient has UC or CD is not important; what matters is that you need to do colonoscopy after 8–10 years of colonic involvement of IBD.
- **Screen for colon cancer after 8–10 years of colon involvement of IBD.**

# Constipation

Make sure you do not miss simple dehydration in the elderly and the need for more fiber in diet.

### Things You Will Be Asked on Rounds

- Use of calcium channel blockers
- Hypothyroidism
- Opiate drug use
- Calcium carbonate replacement
- Tricyclic antidepressant use (anticholinergic)

## Screening for Colon Cancer with Constipation

Nothing is superior to colonoscopy. Stool guaiac lacks specificity and precision. Barium is worthless and impractical. Sigmoidoscopy would miss the 40% of colon cancers that occur proximal to the sigmoid colon.

**Screening Colonoscopy Recommendations by Group**

| Patient Group | Screening Recommendation |
|---|---|
| General population | Age >50 every 10 years |
| One family member | Age >40 or 10 years earlier than family member<br>Every 10 years |
| HNPCC<br>3 family members<br>2 generations<br>1 premature (before 50) | >25 every 1–2 years |
| FAP | Screening sigmoidoscopy every year |

HNPCC = hereditary nonpolyposis colon cancer; FAP = familial adenomatous polyposis

# DIVERTICULAR DISEASE

- Abdominal pain in the left lower quadrant
- Age >50–60
- Diverticulosis diagnosed by endoscopy (colonoscopy)

### Things You Will Be Asked on Rounds

- Blood in the stool
- Fever
- Previous colonoscopy
- Vegetarian diet

## Diverticulitis

Also has:

- Fever
- Leukocytosis
- Acute onset of symptoms
- Diagnosed with CT scan

Avoid scoping diverticulitis because of increased risk of perforation.

### Treatment

There is no specific therapy for diverticulosis. Vegetarians rarely get diverticulosis, so a change in diet to avoid meat and increase fiber will help. Nothing can reverse it.

Diverticulitis is treated with antibiotics such as:

- Ciprofloxacin and metronidazole
- Ceftriaxone and metronidazole

- Ampicillin/sulbactam (Unasyn)
- Piperacillin/tazobactam (Zosyn)
- Any carbapenem (e.g., ertapenem, meropenem, doripenem)

## Cholecystitis

- Right upper quadrant (RUQ) pain and tenderness
- Fever and leukocytosis
- Normal bilirubin and liver function tests in almost all patients
- Ultrasound is best first test
- CT misses some small stones
- Ampicillin/sulbactam (Unasyn)
- Piperacillin/tazobactam (Zosyn)
- Any carbapenem (e.g., ertapenem, meropenem, doripenem)
- Get a surgical evaluation for laparoscopic cholecystectomy

## Ascending Cholangitis

Ascending cholangitis is obstructive jaundice with severe infection of both the biliary tree and the liver. Ascending cholangitis has:

- Biliary tract obstruction causing jaundice
- Increased direct bilirubin
- Alkaline phosphatase and GGTP are elevated.
- AST and ALT may be up as well.

**RUQ pain/tenderness + jaundice = ascending cholangitis**

Don't wait for the "shaking chills," which are a sign of bacteremia!

**Round Saver**

Cholangitis is **much** more severe than cholecystitis!

## Diagnostic Testing and Treatment

In addition to increased liver function tests, diagnosis is confirmed with:

- Ultrasound showing stones and/or ductal dilation
- CT scan
- MRCP (most accurate test of the biliary and pancreatic ductal system)

Mechanical obstruction must be removed/released. ERCP is a therapeutic modality to remove stones and dilate strictures.

Antibiotics are the same as those for cholecystitis. Antibiotics alone will not fix an obstructive stone.

# LIVER DISEASE

Abnormal liver function tests (LFTs) are extremely common with liver disease. For all patients, get the following:

- Repeat LFTs to confirm findings
- Abdominal ultrasound
- Prothrombin time: all clotting factors are made in the liver except factor VIII/vWF
- Albumin
- Hepatitis B and C testing

> **Round Saver**
> Do not have big discussions based on a single abnormal value.

> **Round Saver**
> Make sure you know if liver-toxic medications are being used prior to rounds.

## Things You Will Be Asked on Rounds

- Alcohol use and the medications the patient takes
- The history
    - Call the private doctor! You are going to feel foolish if you present your case as an unknown, only to find the patient has a long history of fully diagnosed chronic hepatitis that he did not tell you about.

**Significance of LFTs**
**(or, "When the XX is abnormal, you should think of YY")**

| Test | Significance |
|---|---|
| AST | Drug toxicity, alcohol |
| ALT | Viral hepatitis |
| Alkaline phosphatase | Biliary tract obstruction<br>Can be from bone too! |
| GGTP | Biliary tract obstruction<br>Goes up immediately after binge drinking |
| Albumin | Synthetic dysfunction of liver<br>Can be down from malnutrition and nephritic syndrome<br>Must be missing 70–80% of liver before it drops |
| Prothrombin time (PT) | Best test of synthetic function of liver<br>Normal PT means liver is working, no matter how high the AST/ALT |

# Viral Hepatitis

If the patient arrives with acute onset of **jaundice and dark urine** (bilirubin in urine), **extreme fatigue**, and **weight loss**, you will not be able to distinguish the specific type of viral hepatitis. Hepatitis makes you feel totally "out of gas." It also shuts off hunger.

## Diagnostic Testing

- Viral hepatitis has markedly elevated direct bilirubin and ALT
- Alkaline phosphatase may be slightly up
- Ultrasound to exclude obstruction
- Biopsy (most accurate test of chronic hepatitis but rarely needed)

Use the following guidelines for specific testing:

| Hepatitis Type | Specific Test |
|---|---|
| A, D, E | IgM acutely, IgG upon resolution |
| C | • Antibody test first<br>• PCR RNA viral load confirms level of activity<br>• Genotype predicts response |
| Acute B | Surface antigen (sAg), e antigen (eAg), core antibody IgM |
| Chronic B | • Persistence of surface antigen >6 months<br>• eAg either positive or negative<br>• Core antibody IgG |
| Vaccine to B | Only surface antibody positive |
| Resolved (past) B | Surface antibody and core antibody IgG |

Hepatitis C PCR RNA indicates whether active infection is present.

## Treatment

The only form of **acute viral hepatitis** that is treated is hepatitis C. We use the following:

**Interferon + ribavirin + boceprevir (or telaprevir)**

Hepatitis C rarely presents in its acute form. Most cases show up years later either on evaluation of abnormal LFTs done for another reason or on development of liver disease. Nevertheless, although rare, this is an excellent opportunity to prevent the development of a chronic disease and potential cirrhosis. Treatment for **chronic hepatitis** generally lasts for 6–12 months.

**Chronic hepatitis C** is treated with the same medications as acute hepatitis C. The adverse effects are:

- Interferon: flu-like symptoms, arthralgia, myalgia, depression
- Ribavirin: anemia

Further management:

- Genotype: determines likelihood of response to treatment
- PCR RNA viral load: determines if a response has occurred
- Biopsy: only way to determine extent of inflammation, fibrosis, or presence of cirrhosis

Note that if viral load is up and you will treat, a biopsy will change little.

**Chronic hepatitis B** uses the same principles of treatment as chronic hepatitis C, though the medications differ. You treat to drive the viral load to undetectable levels. The biopsy determines the extent of disease but adds little if you are going to use medications anyway.

- Monotherapy for hepatitis B
- No genotyping for hepatitis B

- Not clear which drug has better efficacy
    - Lamivudine or
    - Entecavir or
    - Adefovir or
    - Tenofovir or
    - Telbivudine
    - Interferon is by injection and has more adverse effects (flulike symptoms)

Combination therapy is not clearly useful for hepatitis B.

## Cirrhosis

No matter the cause of chronic liver disease, there are a number of common manifestations of cirrhosis. These are based not on the etiology of the disorder but rather on the severity of the disease.

**Manifestations of Cirrhosis and Treatment**

| Manifestation | Treatment |
|---|---|
| Edema | Spironolactone, furosemide |
| Ascites | Spironolactone, furosemide |
| Encephalopathy | Lactulose, rifaximin |
| Low albumin | None |
| High PT/coagulopathy | FFP if bleeding |
| Gynecomastia | None |
| Varices | Propranolol, nadolol<br>Banding if they bleed |
| Splenomegaly | None |
| Hemorrhoids | None |
| Thrombocytopenia | If bleeding, use platelets |

All patients with ascites need a paracentesis to confirm the etiology as portal hypertension causing a transudate and to, at times, exclude **spontaneous bacterial peritonitis (SBP)**. If the ascitic fluid protein level is low (<1 mg/dL), prophylaxis against the first episode of SBP is given with ofloxacin or TMP/SMX.

- Tap (paracentesis) all new onset ascites
- Tap if there is fever or pain/tenderness

**Cell count >250 neutrophils = SBP = cefotaxime (or ceftriaxone)**

One of the reasons to take a sample of all new onset ascitic fluid is to confirm that portal hypertension from cirrhosis is the cause of the ascites. The ascitic fluid or portal hypertension is an extravasation of water based on hydrostatic forces. This is why the ascitic fluid albumin level is low.

**Serum to ascites albumin gradient (SAAG):**

SAAG >1.1

- Portal hypertension
- SBP

SAAG <1.1

- Cancer
- Intra-abdominal infection excluding SBP

## Hemochromatosis

The most common cause of hemochromatosis is a genetic defect resulting in the overabsorption of iron from the duodenum. The iron builds up on the liver, leading to cirrhosis, which is the most common cause of death. Untreated, 20% of patients will develop hepatoma.

Other site manifestations are:

- Joint pain/calcium pyrophosphate deposition disease (pseudogout)
- Diabetes and skin darkening, "bronze diabetes"
- Infertility and pituitary insufficiency

### Diagnostic Testing

Best initial tests:

- Elevated iron and ferritin levels
- Decreased total iron binding capacity (TIBC)

Confirmatory tests:

- Liver biopsy (most accurate)
- HFE gene and MRI can spare the need for liver biopsy

Treatment is phlebotomy (for genetic overabsorbers) or chelators such deferasirox or deferoxamine if overtransfusion is the cause. Phlebotomy removes much more iron than do chelators.

## Wilson's Disease

- Psychosis, paranoia, neurologic abnormalities
- Movement disorder
- Coombs negative hemolysis
- Kayser-Fleischer rings on slit-lamp examination
- Ceruloplasmin level decreased
- Biopsy is most accurate

### Treatment

- Penicillamine
- Zinc
- Trientine

## Primary Biliary Cirrhosis (PBC)

- Women age 40–60
- Itching and xanthelasma
- Alkaline phosphatase elevation
- Anti-mitochondrial antibody
- Treat with ursodeoxycholic acid and sometimes cholestyramine

## Primary Sclerosing Cholangitis (PSC)

- History of inflammatory bowel disease in 80%
- Similar itchy, fatigue to PBC with high alkaline phosphatase
- Bilirubin can be elevated
- MRCP or ERCP is most accurate test
- Treat with ursodeoxycholic acid and sometimes cholestyramine

## Autoimmune Hepatitis

- Young women with positive ANA and increased LFTs
- Elevated anti-smooth muscle antibody
- Anti-liver-kidney microsomal antibody
- Biopsy is most accurate
- Treat with steroids

# ESOPHAGEAL DISORDERS

Many esophageal disorders present with dysphagia and, consequently, weight loss. In the esophagus, barium is fairly good to start with on many disorders you will see in clinic. In the hospital, most disorders are evaluated with endoscopy.

# Esophageal Cancer

Esophageal cancer is strongly associated with progressively worse dysphagia over several weeks to months. "Progressive" means that the difficulty starts first with solid food such as meat and then progresses to soft foods and liquids.

**Round Saver**

Take the history yourself! Double-check notes in chart.

Weight loss is very common with cancer.

**Things You Will Be Asked on Rounds**

- Does food get "stuck" when eating
- Weight loss in the last 6 months
- Pain or difficulty on swallowing
- Fatigue
- Blood in the stool
- Previous smoking history
- Alcohol intake

## Diagnostic Testing

- Upper endoscopy with biopsy
- If cancer seems clear, barium will not be enough
- Chest CT scan evaluates the local extent of disease

## Treatment

- Surgical resection
- Radiation and chemotherapy
- With severe, unresectable cases, a "stent" is placed to push the esophagus open

## Esophageal Spasm

- Chest pain at any time, not just related to eating
- Substernal pain mimics an MI
  - Must do EKG/cardiac enzymes first
- Can be provoked by drinking cold liquids
- Manometry: most accurate test

Treatment is calcium channel blockers and nitrates.

## Achalasia

- Typically, patients are younger (age <40–50) than gastric cancer patients.
- Has no association with alcohol/tobacco.
- Dysphagia occurs with *both* solid foods and liquids at the same time.
- Can be progressive.
- Barium studies show "bird's beak" narrowing.
- Endoscopy shows "tubular esophagus with inability to pass scope into stomach."
- Produces no mucosal abnormality.

The most accurate test is manometry with inadequate relaxation of lower esophageal sphincter (LES).

Treatment is pneumatic dilation by scope, surgical myotomy, or botulinum toxin. Botulinum toxin, however, wears off.

## Esophageal Candidiasis

This disorder is almost exclusively found in patients with AIDS and $CD_4$ cells <100/$mm^3$. A rare person has it from diabetes. Look for a person with AIDS with:

- Odynophagia: pain on swallowing
- Treat with fluconazole 200 mg/day
- Expect a fast response in 1–2 days
- If no response, do endoscopy.

There is not always thrush in the mouth with esophageal disease.

# RINGS AND WEBS

## Schatzki's Ring

- Intermittent dysphagia
- Can be "peptic," meaning from acid coming up into esophagus
- Barium to diagnose distal esophageal narrowing
- Treat with pneumatic dilation

## Plummer Vinson Syndrome

- Proximal, hypopharyngeal web
- Small percentage because squamous cell cancer
- Associated with iron deficiency anemia, but it is **not from GI bleeding**
- Barium to diagnose
- Pneumatic dilation
- Some respond to iron replacement

## Zenker's Diverticulum

- Outpocketing of hypopharyngeal posterior constrictor muscles
- Halitosis from rotting food caught in the diverticulum
- Do NOT do endoscopy
- Do NOT try to pass a nasogastric tube
- Barium to diagnose and surgical resection

## Scleroderma

Look for a patient with scleroderma with severe GERD from an immobile esophagus. Treat the GERD with PPIs. There is no specific therapy simply because it is from scleroderma.

## Mallory-Weiss Tear

Although Mallory-Weiss is a common esophageal disorder, it does not present with dysphagia or odynophagia. Look for a person who develops upper GI bleeding after strenuous vomiting. It occurs from high pressure in the stomach and esophagus.

- Bleeding without dysphagia
- Most resolve spontaneously
- Occasionally an injection of epinephrine is needed to stop the bleeding.

# Hematology 4

## Anemia

The etiology of anemia cannot be determined by its symptoms. Symptoms are determined by the severity of the condition, but only lab testing can determine the etiology. When very severe, anemia presents with syncope and chest pain. Anemia will ultimately lead to death via myocardial ischemia. Look for:

- Fatigue and tiredness
- Shortness of breath, particularly on exertion
- Lightheadedness
- Chest pain and myocardial ischemia

**Round Saver**

Know the EKG and cardiac enzymes in severe anemia!

| Presentation by Severity | |
|---|---|
| **Hematocrit** | **Symptoms** |
| >30–35 | None |
| 25–30 | Fatigue, tiredness |
| 20–25 | Dyspnea |
| 15–20 | Lightheadedness, chest pain |

Symptoms of anemia can easily be confused with those of hypoxia. Do not try to solve anemia symptoms by giving oxygen alone.

## Diagnostic Testing

- Multiple CBC/hematocrit results
  - Is there rapid bleeding? Is CBC stable?
- Platelet count: Multiple cell lines down indicates bone marrow production problem.
- MCV: Cell size is the first clue to etiology.
- Reticulocyte count in the presence of anemia:
  - Low = production defect
  - High = bleeding or hemolysis
- Stool guaiac: Is this GI bleeding?
- PT/INR
  - If it's up, you must give FFP to correct.

Avoid making extensive testing and treatment plans based on a single hematocrit. Repeat any abnormal hematocrit to confirm the results and to determine the trend.

**Round Saver** 

Always repeat the CBC in any anemic patient.

In active bleeding it is utterly impossible to know how fast the blood count is dropping unless you do 2–3 CBCs several hours apart. Know the trend! Hemoglobin level is 1/3 of the hematocrit. This can be used interchangeably with hematocrit.

When **mean corpuscular volume (MCV)** is low (<80 fl), there is a production problem such as iron deficiency. Production problems always take several weeks to develop. When MCV is high (>100 fl), it can be a production problem such as $B_{12}$/folate deficiency, drug or alcohol effect on the marrow, or from blood loss. Reticulocytosis elevates the MCV.

**Reticulocytes** are new, most recently made red cells. Reticulocyte count is low in almost all production problems such as iron, $B_{12}$, or folate deficiency. Chronic diseases also "freeze" the marrow so that reticulocytes are not made. Reticulocyte count is elevated in hemolysis and blood loss. It takes several days for the marrow to raise the reticulocyte count above the usual 1–2%. This means a patient admitted today with an acute GI bleed will not have time to raise the reticulocyte count today.

Correlate findings on smear with the disease.

| Abnormality Seen | Most Likely Cause |
|---|---|
| Fragmented cells: schistocytes, helmet cells | Intravascular hemolysis: TTP/HUS or DIC |
| Target cells | Thalassemia; iron deficiency |
| Bite cells | G6PD deficiency |
| Spherocytes | Hereditary spherocytosis; hemolysis |
| Blasts | Leukemia |
| Teardrop cells | Myelofibrosis |

TTP = thrombotic thrombocytopenic purpura; HUS = hemolytic uremic syndrome; DIC = disseminated intravascular coagulation; G6PD = glucose-6-phosphate dehydrogenase

Heinz bodies are not seen on routine smear.

## Terminology

- RDW = red cell distribution of width
  - Low = all same size
- Anisocytosis = **different sizes** of cells on smear = high RDW
- Poikilocytosis = **different shapes**
- **Bands** = early neutrophils (like a reticulocyte for neutrophils)
- Polychromasia = different colors, usually from reticulocytosis

A high red cell distribution width (RDW) means there are different red cell sizes.

## Treatment

Transfusion of blood always occurs as packed red blood cells (PRBCs). The indication for transfusion depends on the underlying status of the patient:

- Young, healthy patients
  - Wait until hematocrit is at least <20–25, possibly lower. An otherwise healthy person can tolerate this hematocrit during the several days to weeks it takes to produce his or her own new cells.
- Older persons (age >60–70) and those with heart disease
  - Consider PRBCs to keep hematocrit >30%

**How NOT to Kill Your Patient**

Anyone who is symptomatic with shortness of breath or lightheadedness needs to be transfused. Hematocrit should increase by 2–3 points per unit of blood.

### Blood Products

- Packed red cells (standard of care for symptomatic anemia or low hematocrit (<30) in older persons)
- Fresh frozen plasma (FFP) for rapid correction of bleeding from coagulopathy (rarely needed if patient not bleeding)
  - Vitamin K deficiency
  - Warfarin use
  - Liver disease such as in a bleeding alcoholic
  - DIC
- Platelets (transfuse under the following conditions)
  - Patient is bleeding currently and platelet count <50,000/mm$^3$
  - The need is to prevent spontaneous bleeding <10,000/mm$^3$
  - Surgery is needed the same day and platelet count <50,000/mm$^3$

   - Rarely done in idiopathic thrombocytopenic purpura (ITP), even if platelet count is profoundly low. There is little extra clotting ability with 80,000 or 100,000 $mm^3$ platelets than there is at 50,000 or 60,000.
- Cryoprecipitate (never first for anything)
   - Pooled clotting factors, particularly fibrinogen
   - Occasionally used in DIC not controlled with FFP

Whole blood and white cell transfusions are not used in treatment. Whole blood is divided into PRBCs and FFP. White cells simply do not work by the time they get into the recipient.

## Microcytic Anemia

### Presentation

CBC must be obtained to determine if a person has a microcytic anemia (MCV <80 fl). Symptoms such as fatigue and dyspnea are based on severity, not etiology.

#### Things You Will Be Asked on Rounds

- Blood loss, heavy periods (most likely cause: **iron deficiency**)
- Chronic infection, rheumatoid arthritis, cancer, renal failure (most likely cause: **anemia of chronic disease**)
- Alcohol use (most likely cause: **sideroblastic anemia**)
- Very low MCV, few symptoms (most likely cause: **thalassemia**)

## Diagnostic Testing and Treatment

Iron studies are the key to the diagnosis of microcytic anemia. Make sure you get the iron studies (iron, total iron-binding capacity, ferritin) *before* you transfuse blood.

Transfusing 1 unit of blood will invalidate iron studies because the donated blood instantly raises iron levels.

| | Iron Deficiency | Chronic Disease | Sideroblastic | Thalassemia |
|---|---|---|---|---|
| **Iron level** | Low | Low | **HIGH** | Normal |
| **TIBC** | High | **LOW** | Normal | Normal |
| **Ferritin** | **LOW** (normal 30%) | Normal | Normal | Normal |

TIBC = total iron-binding capacity

Specific diagnostic testing and treatment for each disease are as follows.

**Iron deficiency:**

- **Red cell distribution width** (RDW) will be elevated; new cells get smaller as one loses iron.
- Bone marrow (rarely needed): **absence of stainable iron** is the most accurate test.
- **Thrombocytosis** is frequently found.

Treatment is ferrous sulfate 325 mg 3x/day and stool softeners (e.g., colace 100 bid automatically with iron). Tell the patient to expect dark stool and constipation.

**Chronic disease: no specific diagnostic test**

- Low iron
- Low TIBC

Treatment is to fix the underlying disease. Use erythropoietin only for dialysis patients.

**Sideroblastic:**

- Prussian blue stain shows ringed sideroblasts.

Treatment is to stop the toxin (e.g., alcohol, lead, isoniazid). In rare cases, vitamin $B_6$ is helpful.

**Thalassemia:**

- Hemoglobin electrophoresis
  - Beta thalassemia: decreased hemoglobin A (HbA)
    - Increased HbF
    - Increased HbA2
  - Alpha thalassemia:
    - Normal electrophoresis
    - Needs genetic studies for clear diagnosis
    - 3-gene deletion: hemoglobin H (4 beta chains)

There is no treatment for the thalassemia trait.

## Macrocytic Anemia (MCV >100 fl)

There are many causes of large red cells ("macrocytosis"), but very few causes of megaloblastic anemia ("hypersegmentation"). Hypersegmentation is defined as >4 lobes per neutrophil. $B_{12}$ or folate deficiency can cause hypersegmentation, as can antimetabolite medications such as azathioprine or 6-MP.

Phenytoin causes folate deficiency.

**Macrocytosis:**

- Vitamin $B_{12}$ or folate deficiency
- Alcohol

> **Round Saver**
>
> Look like a star! Know that megaloblastic anemia = hypersegmentation.

- Medications: zidovudine (AZT), hydroxyurea, azathioprine, 6-MP
- Hypothyroidism
- Liver disease
- Phenytoin (leads to folate deficiency)

**Round Saver**

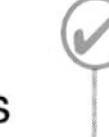

See the smear. It is the only way to find hypersegmentation.

# Vitamin $B_{12}$ Deficiency

## Presentation

Look for a person with fatigue, shortness of breath, and possibly lightheadedness of anemia with an elevated MCV. The first step is to look at the peripheral smear for hypersegmentation. You do not have to have neurological manifestations to have $B_{12}$ deficiency. You can have the neurological manifestations alone or hematological manifestations alone or both together.

Any defect of the neurologic system is possible:

- Peripheral neuropathy (most common)
- Loss of position and vibratory sense (much less common than peripheral neuropathy)
- Dementia (least common)

Neurologic abnormalities are reversible if they are minor and of short duration.

## Etiology

- Pernicious anemia: autoimmune event against gastric lining
- Nutritional deficiency
- Pancreatic insufficiency
- Crohn's disease, celiac disease, or anything else that damages the terminal ileum

### Diagnostic Testing and Treatment

- Smear: hypersegmentation
- Elevated indirect bilirubin and LDH with low reticulocyte count from "ineffective erythropoiesis"
- Vitamin $B_{12}$ level: may be falsely normal in 30%
- Methylmalonic acid elevated only in $B_{12}$ deficiency
- Anti-intrinsic factor and antiparietal cell antibodies positive in pernicious anemia

Macro-ovalocytes are common on smear.

Replace vitamin $B_1$2 with an intramuscular injection at first and then orally. Extremely rapid cellular production can use up all the potassium in the blood. Watch out for hypokalemia.

## Folate Deficiency

Folate deficiency is caused by nutritional deficiency, especially in combination with increased cell turnover such as in psoriasis or chronic hemolysis with sickle cell disease.

- Macrocytic anemia with hypersegmented neutrophils
- Neurologic abnormalities are never seen.
- Do the peripheral smear and check the folic acid level.
- Methylmalonic acid level will be normal.

Replace folate orally and look for immediate response in cell counts over subsequent days.

## Hemolytic Anemia

Make sure the following tests are done on every patient suspected of hemolysis:

- Reticulocyte count (increased)

- Indirect bilirubin and LDH (increased)
- Haptoglobin (decreased)
- Peripheral smear with intravascular hemolysis and sickle cell (abnormal)

Aside from a smear that shows sickled cells, the tests above will not distinguish the type of hemolysis at hand. Clues to specific types of hemolysis are as follows:

| Things You Will Be Asked on Rounds | Diagnosis | Confirmatory Test |
|---|---|---|
| Pain in back, chest, thighs | **Sickle cell** | Smear, electrophoresis |
| Penicillin, CLL, lymphoma, SLE | **Autoimmune (warm IgG)** | Coombs test |
| Pain in nose, ears, fingers | **Cold agglutinin** | IgM cold agglutinins |
| Thrombocytopenia, increased BUN/creatinine | **HUS/TTP** | Fragmented cells on smear<br>Normal PT/aPTT/INR |
| Current infection, sulfa drug | **G6PD deficiency** | Heinz bodies, bite cells, G6PD level after 2 months |
| Previous episodes, big spleen, bilirubin gallstones | **Hereditary spherocytosis** | Increased MCHC, osmotic fragility |
| Dark morning urine, clots, pancytopenia | **Paroxysmal nocturnal hemoglobinuria (PNH)** | Hemoglobinuria, CD55/59 |

CLL: chronic lymphocytic leukemia; G6PD: glucose-6-phosphate dehydrogenase; MCHC: mean corpuscular hemoglobin concentration; HUS: hemolytic uremic syndrome; TTP: thrombotic thrombocytopenic purpura

### Intravascular Hemolysis

- Cells are destroyed in blood vessels.
- Fragmented cells: schistocytes, helmet cells
- TTP, HUS, DIC
- Can give hemoglobin in urine!
- No hemolysis will give bilirubin in the urine.
- Indirect bilirubin is attached to albumin.

**Round Saver**

*Extra*vascular = spleen (or liver).

## Sickle Cell Disease

On a medicine rotation it is extremely unlikely that you will encounter a person being diagnosed with sickle cell for the first time. Patients have a lifelong history of the following:

- Chronic hemolysis
- Hospitalizations for painful sickle crises several times a year
- Long-term folic acid replacement
- Hydroxyurea use for 4+ crises per year

**Round Saver**

Hypoxia, dehydration, and infection lead to pain crisis but are not essential.

**Things You Will Be Asked on Rounds**

Sickle cell disease

- Pain in chest, back, and thighs
- Dehydration, fever, infection
- Dyspnea: hypoxia causes sickling
- Visual disturbance, priapism, signs of stroke: these need immediate transfusion

## Diagnostic Testing

These tests are critical for sickle cell diagnosis.

- WBC count: higher than usual = infection
- Reticulocyte count: low = *Parvovirus*
- If fever is present, do chest x-ray, UA, and blood culture.

Hemoglobin electrophoresis should be done at least once to confirm the diagnosis.

## Treatment

- Oxygen, fluids, pain medication
- If fever is present or leukocytosis is higher than usual, give an antibiotic such as ceftriaxone, levofloxacin, or moxifloxacin immediately.
- Folic acid
- Vaccination for *Haemophilus*, meningococcus, and pneumococcus (if not already documented)
- Parvovirus will "freeze" the marrow at the level or pronormoblast and stop all reticulocyte production. Look for a sudden drop in hematocrit >3–4 points over several days.
  - Sickle crisis, by itself, should **not** drop the hematocrit >3–4 points.
  - Parvovirus eliminates reticulocytes first.
  - PCR-DNA is more accurate than IgM against parvovirus.
  - Treat with IVIG
  - Make sure it is not simple folic acid deficiency first.

**Round Saver**

Fever and increased leukocytosis require immediate antibiotics.

## Sickle Cell Trait (Heterozygous or AS Disease)

- Hematologically normal
- Smear and CBC: normal
- Only manifestation is renal
- Ask about hematuria, frequent urine infections, and dehydration
- AS gives renal/urinary concentrating defect

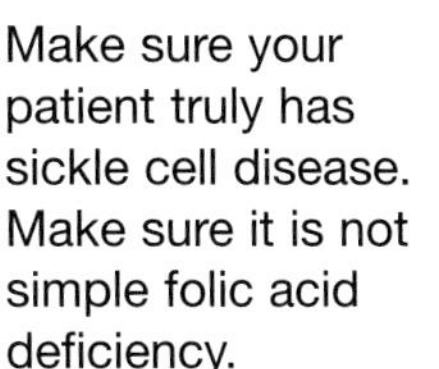


There is no specific therapy for AS disease.

## Treatment

Disease-specific treatment of hemolysis is advised as follows:

| Diagnosis | Treatment |
|---|---|
| **Autoimmune (warm IgG) hemolytic anemia** | • Prednisone, methylprednisolone<br>• IVIG for severe cases<br>• Splenectomy for recurrent cases |
| **Cold agglutinin disease** | • Rituximab<br>• Steroids do NOT work |
| **HUS/TTP** | • Plasmapheresis for severe<br>• Do NOT transfuse platelets!!!<br>• Do NOT treat *E. coli* |
| **G6PD deficiency** | • No specific therapy |
| **Hereditary spherocytosis** | • Chronic folic acid replacement<br>• Splenectomy in severe cases |
| **Paroxysmal nocturnal hemoglobinuria (PNH)** | • Glucocorticoids<br>• Eculizumab (anti-complement anti-body) |

## COAGULATION DISORDERS

The most important issues in the assessment of a bleeding patient are:

- Is the bleeding related to clotting factor disorder or platelets?
- How much blood has been lost?

The issues of blood loss volume and indications for transfusion are covered at the beginning of the anemia section. Basically, transfuse all symptomatic persons and older persons who have both heart disease and hematocrit <30%.

Determine the type of bleeding **before** you look at the blood tests.

| Platelet vs. Factor-Type Bleeding | |
|---|---|
| **Platelet Disorder (low count or dysfunction)** | **Clotting Factor Disorder** |
| Superficial bleeding | Deep bleeding |
| • Epistaxis<br>• Petechiae, purpura<br>• Gums, gingiva<br>• Menstrual | • Hemarthrosis (joint)<br>• Hematoma (muscle) |

Bleeding of the GI tract or CNS can be caused by either a platelet or clotting factor disorder.

## Von Willebrand's Disease

Look for:

- Platelet-type bleeding and a normal platelet count
- Worse with the use of aspirin
- Lifelong, recurrent, and often with a family history

### Diagnostic Testing

Von Willebrand's can be caused by a deficiency of von Willebrand's factor (VWF) or by a defect in its function. You should order both a level of VWF and the ristocetin cofactor assay, which test the function of VWF.

- VWF is synonymous with factor VIII antigen
- 50% will have an elevated aPTT because defective VWF destabilizes the factor VIII coagulant, which is the hemophilia A factor.
- Bleeding time is rarely done. In this test, you cut the patient and time how long it takes to stop bleeding.

### Treatment

- Initial therapy is DDAVP. (desmopressin)
- If no response, replace factor VIII.

> **Round Saver**
>
> Factor VIII contains VWF!!

## Immune (or Idiopathic) Thrombocytopenic Purpura (ITP)

- Profoundly low platelet count
- Bleeding when <10,000–20,000/mcL
- Normal-size spleen
- Normal WBC count and differential

ITP is a diagnosis of exclusion. There is no test to prove one has the disease. Bone marrow biopsy is done to exclude a production defect when the diagnosis is not clear from the history. However, do not delay treatment waiting for bone marrow.

> **Round Saver** 
> Antiplatelet antibodies do NOT help!

### Treatment

When a person presents with isolated thrombocytopenia and a normal-sized spleen, do not delay therapy to wait for testing results.

- Prednisone is the best initial therapy.
- If recurrences are frequent after steroids have been stopped, do a splenectomy.
  - After splenectomy, recurrences can be managed with romiplostim or eltrombopag.
- Life-threatening bleeding needs IVIG.

> **Round Saver** 
> Give IVIG for intracranial or major GI bleeding.

## Warfarin Overdose, Vitamin K Deficiency, and Liver Disease

These disorders present identically, with elevations in PT, aPTT, and INR.

- Fresh frozen plasma (FFP) is the fastest way to reverse the effect of warfarin and stop bleeding.
  - If there is bleeding with any of these disorders, use FFP immediately.
  - FFP lasts only for a few hours or a day.

- With vitamin K deficiency, also replace vitamin K.
- With warfarin overdose, the decision to replace vitamin K must be based on whether you want to continue the warfarin later as therapy, at a lower intensity.
    - If warfarin is no longer needed, replace vitamin K as well.

**Round Saver**

FFP is the fastest way to reverse warfarin overdose if bleeding.

## Disseminated Intravascular Coagulopathy (DIC)

DIC presents with bleeding related to both platelet loss as well as clotting factor deficiency. This is why you will see elevated PT and aPTT, as well as low platelets. You do not have to give platelets if platelet count >50,000.

DIC does not happen in routine admissions. Look for a major disease such as sepsis, cancer, leukemia, or amniotic fluid embolus.

### Diagnostic Testing

Signs of hemolysis are common in DIC: increased LDH, reticulocytes, and indirect bilirubin.

- Elevated PT, aPTT, and INR
- Decreased platelets
- Elevated D-dimers and fibrin split products
- Decreased fibrinogen
- Fragmented cells (schistocytes and helmet cells) on smear

## Treatment

- Replace FFP.
- Give platelets when the count is <50,000 and the patient is bleeding.
- Heparin is not useful.

## Heparin-Induced Thrombocytopenia (HIT)

HIT is defined as >50% drop in platelets with the use of any amount of heparin. It typically starts to take effect a few days after heparin has been used.

- Enoxaparin (LMW) has less risk of HIT, but not zero risk.
- Do **not** wait for antiplatelet factor 4 antibodies or the serotonin release assay to stop the heparin.
- If full-dose anticoagulation is needed (e.g., PE), use argatroban or lepirudin.
- HIT causes *both* venous and arterial thrombosis.

**Round Saver** 

You can't just switch to low molecular weight heparin after getting HIT on IV heparin.

**Round Saver** 

Even tiny amounts of heparin can cause HIT, as with a flush or DVT prophylaxis.

# CLOTTING FACTOR DEFICIENCIES

## Hemophilia

Look for:

- Joint bleeding delayed 1–2 days after trauma. The primary hemostatic plug is with platelets. This dissolves if fibrin is not produced to solidify the plug.
- Increased aPTT with a normal PT
- Correction of the aPTT to normal upon mixing it with normal plasma

> **Round Saver**
>
> Mixing study corrects aPTT to normal with deficiency, but not with clotting factor inhibitor.

Treat mild disease with DDAVP and severe disease with factor VIII or IX replacement as needed.

## Factor XI and XII Deficiencies

Both factor XI and factor XII deficiencies produce elevated aPTT with normal PT. Both correct to normal when mixing 50:50 with normal plasma.

- Factor XII deficiency never bleeds.
- Factor XI deficiency will bleed with unusual circumstances such as trauma or surgery. When bleeding is associated with factor XI deficiency, treat with FFP.

## Hypercoagulable States/Thrombophilia

Deep venous thrombosis (DVT) and pulmonary emboli (PE) are common diagnoses. DVT is treated almost exclusively as an outpatient with subcutaneous injection of LMW heparin followed by warfarin for 6 months. Target INR for both disorders is 2–3.

Evaluation for thrombophilia is not necessary during the acute episode of thrombosis. The only thrombophilic state that alters management is antiphospholipid (APL) syndrome, sometimes called anticardiolipin antibody and lupus anticoagulant. This is because the APL syndrome is the only one in which we may treat lifelong with even a single clot.

Although the most common cause of thrombophilia is factor V Leiden mutation, it does not change the intensity or the duration of anticoagulation. The same is true of protein C or S deficiency and antithrombin deficiency.

# HEMATOLOGICAL MALIGNANCIES

## Chronic Lymphocytic Leukemia (CLL)

CLL is the most common hematologic malignancy in persons age >60. Look for an older person who possibly has splenomegaly or adenopathy.

### Diagnostic Testing

CLL has no single clear diagnostic blood test.

- High WBC count (>20,000–30,000/mcL)
- >80–90% lymphocytes
- Normal appearance on smear
- Anemia and thrombocytopenia in severe disease

## Treatment

Early stage CLL (0–1) needs no treatment. Advanced-stage disease (2–4) and those with symptoms need treatment.

| Stage | Symptoms | Treatment |
|---|---|---|
| 0 | lymphocytosis only | no treatment |
| 1 | adenopathy | no treatment |
| 2 | splenomegaly | fludarabine |
| 3 | anemia | fludarabine |
| 4 | thrombocytopenia | fludarabine |

Anemia and thrombocytopenia may be from autoimmune antibodies. If this is the case, treat with steroids, not chemotherapy. Chlorambucil is an alternative to fludarabine in those not young or stable enough to use fludarabine.

- Rituximab or cyclophosphamide is sometimes added to treatment for CLL.
- IVIG is used if recurrent infections occur.

# Chronic Myelogenous Leukemia (CML)

Look for:

- WBC elevated >20,000–30,000
- >80–90% neutrophils
- Splenomegaly and early satiety
- Increased infections and fatigue
- Itching from basophils

## Diagnostic Testing

- *BCR-ABL* PCR of peripheral blood (Philadelphia [Ph] chromosome)
- Low leukocyte alkaline phosphatase (LAP) score (rarely used)
    - Attendings often ask about LAP score.
- Normal-appearing smear

## Treatment

- Tyrosine kinase inhibitor: imatinib, dasatinib, nilotinib
- Bone marrow transplant is the only way to cure the disease, but is rarely needed.

# Pancytopenia

All 3 cell lines can be suppressed by:

- Primary or metastatic cancer invading the bone marrow
- Infections such as TB, fungi, hepatitis B or C, HIV, CMV, or EBV
- Autoimmune diseases: SLE
- $B_{12}$ or folate deficiency
- Myelodysplastic syndrome (MDS)
- Drug effect: sulfa, phenytoin, carbamazepine, propylthiouracil
- Alcohol
- PNH

## Diagnostic Testing

Exclude all these diseases by blood tests with the admission orders. If nothing is found, pancytopenia needs bone marrow biopsy to determine the diagnosis.

> **Round Saver**
>
> Tell your attending—**before** you are asked—that you think bone marrow is needed.

# Aplastic Anemia

Aplastic anemia is a pancytopenia of unclear etiology. When there is no identifiable etiology for pancytopenia, it is from a type of autoimmune disorder in which a patient's killer T-cells attack the rest of the bone marrow to suppress it.

## Treatment

- Allogeneic bone marrow transplantation (age <50 with a match)
- Age >50 or no match possible:
  - Cyclosporine
  - Antithymocyte globulin (ATG)
  - Tacrolimus or sirolimus

# Myelodysplastic Syndrome

Myelodysplastic syndrome (MDS) is one of the causes of pancytopenia, which cannot be detected until after the bone marrow biopsy has been done. There is absolutely nothing unique in the history, physical, or possible symptoms that can tell you, for sure, that the person has MDS.

Look for an older patient who presents with:

- Fatigue from anemia
- Bleeding when platelets <30,000–50,000/$mm^3$
- Infection

**Round Saver**

MDS is a laboratory diagnosis.

## Diagnostic Testing

- Pancytopenia
- Increased MCV with normal $B_{12}$/folate levels

- Bilobed neutrophils (Pelger-Huet cell)
- Ringed sideroblasts on Prussian blue stain
- 5q deletion
- Variable number of blasts present (the greater the number, the worse the disease)

**Round Saver**

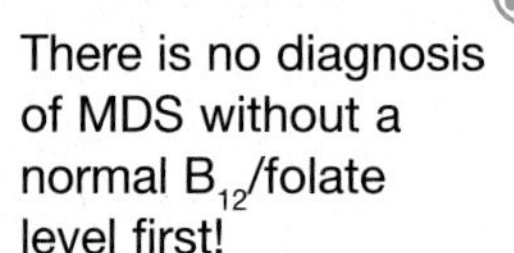

There is no diagnosis of MDS without a normal $B_{12}$/folate level first!

### Treatment

- Supportive with transfusion and erythropoietin
- Lenalidomide
- Azacytidine

## Myelofibrosis

Myelofibrosis is pancytopenia in association with:

- Teardrop-shaped red cells on smear
- Reticulin fibers on bone marrow biopsy
- Large spleen from extramedullary hematopoiesis
    - Red cell production switches to the spleen because the reticulin fibers make it impossible for the cells to be produced in the marrow.

Treat with lenalidomide. Do bone marrow transplantation if patient is young enough (age <50).

## Hairy Cell Leukemia

- Age 50–60
- Pancytopenia
- Splenomegaly

- No teardrop cells or reticulin fibers on marrow biopsy
- Tartrate-resistant acid phosphatase (TRAP)
- "Hairy" projections on the white cells

Treat hairy cell leukemia with cladribine.

## Polycythemia Vera

Polycythemia vera (p. vera) is a red cell cancer sometimes associated with an elevated platelet and WBC count. P. vera presents with:

- Hematocrit >55–60%
- Thrombosis or bleeding
- Dyspnea
- Facial "plethora"
- Fatigue
- Headache, blurred vision

### Diagnostic Testing

To diagnose p. vera, hypoxia must be excluded as the cause of the red cell elevation. Hypoxia also causes microcytic (MCV <80) erythrocytosis.

- JAK2 mutation 95%
- Vitamin $B_{12}$ elevated

### Treatment

- Phlebotomy
- Hydroxyurea helps bring down the red cell count in some cases.

## Essential Thrombocythemia

Essential thrombocythemia (ET) is cancer of platelets and megakaryocytes.

- Platelet count >1,000,000
- Thrombosis or bleeding
- JAK2 mutation

Treat ET with hydroxyurea. Anagrelide is sometimes used. In those with thrombosis, use aspirin.

> **Round Saver**
> Reactive thrombocytosis rarely hits 1 million platelets.

## Acute Leukemia

### Presentation

Acute leukemia presents with signs of pancytopenia even though WBC count is elevated in 30% of patients. This is because, by definition, acute leukemia is characterized by white cells that are "blasts," and blasts simply do not function. These blasts crowd out the rest of the marrow, bringing down both the red cell and platelet count.

> **Round Saver**
> It is possible that no one else but you will notice the life-threatening disease!

Look for:

- Bleeding
- Infection
- Fatigue

### Diagnostic Testing

- Examine the peripheral smear for blasts.
- Refer to hematology for bone marrow biopsy.
- Exclude Auer rods.
- Flow cytometry (cell sorting) makes definitive diagnosis.
- Myeloperoxidase, Auer rods, and nonspecific esterase are not as important as flow cytometry.

### Treatment

- Transfuse blood and platelets as needed.
- Daunorubicin and cytosine arabinoside (Ara-C) for AML
- Add all-trans-retinoic acid (ATRA) for M3 promyelocytic leukemia.
- Bone marrow transplant if cytogenetic anomalies indicate a high risk of relapse.

## Leukostasis Reaction

Leukostasis occurs when the WBC count is so high that it leads to sludging in the blood vessels of the brain, lungs, and eyes. When WBC >100,000/mcL, blockage of the flow of blood can result in tissue hypoxia. Look for:

- Myelogenous leukemia, either acute or chronic (lymphocytes are generally too small to cause leukostasis)
- Dyspnea
- Priapism
- Confusion

Treat with leukapheresis and hydroxyurea to bring down the cell count. Hydrate the patient.

## Lymphoma

Look for:

- Lymph nodes that are very large
- Lymphadenopathy that is NOT red, warm, or tender
- Splenomegaly (common)
- Hodgkin's (localized to stage I or II in 80–90%)
- Non-Hodgkin's (stage III or IV in 80–90%)
- Ask about fever, weight loss, and sweating at night

**Staging** is the same for both Hodgkin's disease (HD) and non-Hodgkin's lymphoma (NHL):

| | |
|---|---|
| Stage I | One group of nodes |
| Stage II | Two or more groups, but on the same side of the diaphragm |
| Stage III | Both sides of the diaphragm |
| Stage IV | Diffuse |

### Diagnostic Testing

A needle sample cannot tell whether the lymphocytes are lymphoma.

- Excisional lymph node biopsy (best initial test)
    - Needle biopsy is not adequate for lymphoma.
- Elevated LDH is expected.
- CT scan of the chest, abdomen, and pelvis
- Bone marrow biopsy

**Staging evaluation:** The point of the tests, which determine the stage of lymphoma, is to determine the treatment. Localized disease to 1 or 2 lymph node groups needs less chemotherapy than more extensive disease. Extensive disease (stage III or IV) or with "B" symptoms of fever, >10% weight loss, or night sweats is always treated with combination chemotherapy.

If you have disease that is local but give extensive chemotherapy, the patient develops unnecessary adverse effects. If you radiate local lesions in the neck but there is disease extended into the pelvis, the patient will die of untreated lymphoma. Radiate local, chemo widespread.

### Treatment

For Hodgkin's disease, use ABVD (adriamycin, bleomycin, vinblastine, dacarbazine).

- Adriamycin can cause cardiomyopathy.
- Bleomycin can cause lung fibrosis.
- Vinblastine can cause peripheral neuropathy.

For non-Hodgkin's lymphoma, use CHOP-R (cyclophosphamide, hydroxyadriamycin, oncovin/vincristine, prednisone, rituximab).

- Cyclophosphamide can cause hemorrhagic cystitis.
- Vincristine can cause peripheral neuropathy.

## Myeloma

Myeloma kills through infection and renal failure. Look for someone with bone pain from a pathologic fracture, i.e., a fracture in which the bone breaks under "normal" use. The most common sites of fracture in myeloma are ribs, vertebra, and wrist.

Also look for:

- Anemia (normocytic)
- Hypercalcemia
- High serum protein level
- Frequent infections and renal insufficiency

## Diagnostic Testing

The most common presentation of myeloma is bone pain. Thus, you should expect to see lytic lesions on x-ray of the affected bones. High serum protein will need a serum protein electrophoresis (SPEP), which will show a monoclonal (one type) of immunoglobulin in the IgG or IgA class. When this "monoclonal" spike is called an "M-spike," it means it is made against a single antigen. It does not mean it is an IgM.

- Increased BUN/creatinine
- Beta-2 microglobulin
- Hyperuricemia
- Bence-Jones proteins seen on urine immunoelectrophoresis (not seen on standard urinalysis)
- Smear can show "rouleaux" or red cells in "rolls"
- >10% plasma cells on bone marrow biopsy

> **Round Saver**
>
> M-spike alone is not myeloma.

The most specific test for myeloma is increased plasma cells on marrow.

## Treatment

Myeloma therapy is one of the agents to start, or a combination of:

- Lenalidomide
- Melphalan
- Steroids
- Bortezomib

At this time, it is not clear which drug or which combination to start with. In those age <70, autologous stem cell transplant is highly effective.

## Monoclonal Gammopathy of Unknown Significance (MGUS)

MGUS is 50–100x more common than myeloma. MGUS presents with:

- High total serum protein
- Age >60–70
- **No symptoms**
- Monoclonal spike usually in IgG class
- Every other test is normal (normal calcium, CBC, and uric acid)
- No bone lesions

There is no treatment for MGUS. About 1% of cases transform into myeloma.

# Waldenström's Macroglobulinemia

- Similar to myeloma but with IgM
- SPEP shows the IgM
- No bone lesions
- No hypercalcemia

## Presentation

Look for hyperviscosity because the IgM is much bigger than an IgG. Also watch for:

- Dyspnea
- Confusion
- Blurry vision with "sausage vessels" on fundoscopy

To treat, use plasmapheresis to remove hyperviscosity. Alkylating agents such as fludarabine, melphalan, and chlorambucil can decrease plasma cells.

# Infectious Diseases 5

## Fever Evaluation

Temperature <38°C (100.4°F) is **not** a fever.

- Persistent fever is more dangerous than a single elevation.
- Typically, normal rectal temperature can be 0.5°C (1°F) higher than oral.
- Fever + hypotension/tachycardia = **danger.**
- Fever + hypotension/tachycardia + acidosis + confusion = sepsis = **worse danger.**
- Fever + hypotension/tachycardia/acidosis/confusion + renal + lung failure = severe sepsis = **death.**

> **Round Saver**
> 99.7°F is **not** a fever.

When evaluating fever, it is important to know *what you should not do*. Beware of what you see your resident do!

Aside from blood culture, **do not send a culture without evidence of infection**. This is hard for students to understand. For example, sputum that grows *Staphylococcus* is not automatically pneumonia from *Staphylococcus*. Instead, it can be one of the following:

- Contaminant from a sloppy sample collection
- Colonization of the mouth
- Colonization from an endotracheal or tracheostomy tube

### How NOT to Kill Your Patient

If your febrile patient **has low BP (systolic <90 mmHg)** and **confusion or metabolic acidosis**, stop reading this book and get your resident! This is sepsis and the patient needs 500–1,000 mL of saline, blood cultures, and IV antibiotics stat!

Everyone with unexplained fever needs:

- Blood cultures: 2 sets from different sites
- Chest x-ray (CXR)
- Urinalysis (UA)

This is expressly for those in whom the site of infection is not clear. If a person presents with an obvious skin infection from cellulitis causing fever, for instance, there is no need to get a UA. Your experience in the hospital will be:

### Round Saver

The word "spike" is not as precise as a number. With fever, use numbers.

1. How high is a temperature that is considered "fever"? (answer: >38°C/100.4°F)
2. How far do you go in testing to be sure fever is not dangerous?

## Specific Cultures That Are Useless

Cultures in the circumstances below are actually **worse than useless**. They generate abnormal cultures without evidence of disease, leading to unnecessary antibiotic use.

1. Do not do urine culture without WBCs on UA.
2. Do not do sputum culture without a new infiltrate on chest x-ray and sputum production.
3. Do not swab skin ulcers and send for culture. **For any ulcer on which you swab the surface, something will grow**. Ulcers

of diabetic feet and legs will always grow organisms, but that does not mean those are the organisms that led to the infection.

Adverse consequences of unnecessary cultures are:

- Prolonged stay in the hospital, administering antibiotics for no benefit
- *Clostridium difficile* colitis/antibiotic-associated diarrhea
- Colonization or infection now pushed into resistant organisms

Do not treat wound or urine "colonization" with antibiotics.

## Leukocytosis

An elevated WBC count on CBC ("leukocytosis") should be evaluated or treated the same way as fever.

- Look for/ask about a clear cause or site of infection.
  - Urine, lung, and skin are the most common.
- Do 2 blood cultures, chest x-ray, and urinalysis.
- Do not do a urine culture unless there are WBCs in urine.
- Do not do a sputum culture unless there is a new infiltrate on CXR and sputum production.

This means that the only culture to be done automatically in the evaluation of fever is blood culture. This means waiting for the results of the UA before sending the urine culture. You may hear the term "pan-culture," or worse, you may see residents and attendings requesting automatic cultures of urine and sputum on every patient with fever as, "Get pan-culture."

**Round Saver**

Anyone saying "Get pan-culture" is **wrong**! Do not learn from that person.

Urine culture that grows yeast or *E. coli* with no evidence of infection such as WBCs on UA should not be treated. The only exception here is pregnancy, for which treatment should be done. *E. coli* growing from urine without WBCs or dysuria can be the result of:

- Colonization of a urinary (Foley) catheter
- Contamination on urine collection
  - "Clean catch" urine can be very hard to obtain in bedbound patients, particularly women and those with dementia/confusion.

Blood culture can be contaminated with skin bacteria (flora) from inadequate preparation. If the blood culture grows an organism, you need to be sure it is a true infection and not contamination. If the same organism can be grown from multiple sites, that strongly supports a genuine infection. **Take blood cultures from multiple sites.**

## Summary of Fever Evaluation

- Temperature <38°C/100.4°F is not a fever. Do not do anything.
- If patient is truly febrile, find local site first (urine/lung/skin/wounds, etc.)
- Taking blood cultures (2), UA, and CXR is the only routine "fever evaluation in those without localizing source."
- If there is no evidence of infection, do not culture it.

The only "routine" culture for a febrile patient is blood culture.

# Sepsis

While obtaining a culture without evidence of infection is potentially harmful, it is even more dangerous to withhold antibiotics when a person has evidence of sepsis. Suspect sepsis when there is:

- Fever + hypotension + tachycardia
- Metabolic acidosis (pH <7.2) with decreased serum bicarbonate
- Increased anion gap
- Respiratory alkalosis ($pCO_2$ <35) to compensate
- Leukocytosis or low WBC (less important than acidosis and hypotension)

With sepsis, you should order blood culture, UA, and CXR. **Administer antibiotics immediately**, without waiting for results; you cannot wait 1–2 days for blood culture results if the person is septic.

Renal and hepatic failure plus CNS disturbance will lead to a **more severe sepsis**.

## Treatment

Treatment for sepsis is empiric, i.e., treating before you know the results of the culture. There is no one single treatment.

Start with vancomycin plus 1 of the following:

- Piperacillin/tazobactam (Zosyn) or ticarcillin/clavulanic acid (Timentin)
- Carbapenem (meropenem or doripenem or imipenem)
- Cefepime or ceftazidime

For severe sepsis, add a second Gram-negative agent such as:

- Fluoroquinolone (Ciprofloxacin or Levofloxacin)
- Monobactam (Aztreonam)
- Aminoglycoside (Gentamicin, Amikacin, Tobramycin)

# Introduction to Antibiotics

| Antibiotics for Gram-Negative Bacilli (Rods) | | | | | |
|---|---|---|---|---|---|
| **Fluoroquinolone** | **Penicillin** | **Cephalosporin** | **Aminoglycoside** | **Monobactam** | **Carbapenem** |
| Ciprofloxacin<br>Levofloxacin<br>Moxifloxacin<br>Gemifloxacin | Piperacillin<br>Ticarcillin | Cef***triaxone***<br>Cefo***taxime***<br>Cef***epime***<br>Cef***tazidime*** | Gentamicin<br>Tobramycin<br>Amikacin | Aztreonam | Meropenem<br>Doripenem<br>Imipenem<br>**Erta**penem |
| Cipro does not cover pneumococcus | Not used without beta-lactamase inhibitor | Ceftriaxone #1 for pneumococcus | Never use as single agents | No cross-reaction with penicillin | **Erta** does not cover *Pseudomonas* |

With penicillin allergy, use cephalosporin in cases of rash alone.

| Antibiotics by Organism/Disease Group | | | |
|---|---|---|---|
| **Organism** | **Staphylococcus/ Streptococcus** | **Gram-Negative Rods** | **Anaerobes** |
| **Diseases Caused** | Bone/heart/skin/joint | Urine/gastrointestinal/liver | Abdominal/abscesses |
| **Antibiotics** | IV: oxacillin, nafcillin, cefazolin<br><br>Oral: dicloxacillin, cephalexin | Ceftriaxone, cefotaxime, cefepime<br>quinolones, carbapenems, aminoglycoside, aztreonam | GI: metronidazole<br>carbapenems,<br>beta-lactam/lactamase<br><br>Respiratory: clindamycin<br>beta-lactam/lactamase |

Gram-negative rods = *E. coli, Enterobacter, Pseudomonas, Citrobacter, Klebsiella, Proteus, Serratia, Morganella;* Staphylococcus = aureus; Streptococcus = pyogenes

Tigecycline covers MRSA and Gram-negative rods.

| MRSA | |
|---|---|
| **Severe: Lung, Heart, CNS, Bacteremia** | **Minor Local: Skin** |
| • Vancomycin<br>• Linezolid (thrombocytopenia)<br>• Daptomycin (CPK elevation)<br>• Tigecycline<br>• Ceftaroline | • TMP/SMZ<br>• Clindamycin<br>• Doxycycline<br>• Linezolid |

Daptomycin is not effective in the lungs. Ceftaroline is the only cephalosporin that covers MRSA.

Beta-lactam/beta-lactamase medications:

- Ampicillin/sulbactam (Unasyn)
- Amoxacillin/clavulanic acid (Augmentin)
- Piperacillin/tazobactam (Zosyn)
- Ticarcillin/clavulanic acid (Timentin)

The beta-lactam/beta-lactamase medications all cover:

- Streptococcus
- Anaerobes
- Most Gram-negative rods (e.g., *E. coli, Proteus, Klebsiella, Enterobacter*)
    - Piperacillin and ticarcillin also cover ***Pseudomonas***

The beta-lactamase inhibitor:

- Adds Staphylococcus coverage
- Expands Gram-negative rod coverage

**Round Saver**

When there is penicillin allergy, always ask the patient to clarify the specific allergy: what happened?

## Antibiotics Safe in Pregnancy

- Penicillins: all of them
- Cephalosporins: all of them
- Aztreonam
- Carbapenems
- Nitrofurantoin
- Metronidazole
- Azithromycin

## Adverse Effects of Antibiotics

The cross-reaction between penicillin and cephalosporin is very limited. Many patients lose their penicillin allergy over time. If the penicillin allergy was only a rash, you can safely use cephalosporins. If the allergy was anaphylaxis, avoid both the cephalosporins and carbapenems. It is completely safe to use aztreonam with any type of penicillin allergy.

**Round Saver**

If rash was the patient's only reaction to penicillin, cephalosporins are safe.

| Antibiotic | Adverse Effect/Caution |
|---|---|
| Daptomycin | • CPK elevation<br>• Not effective in lung |
| Metronidazole | • No alcohol! Causes vomiting<br>• Metal taste<br>• CNS disturbance |
| Imipenem | • Seizures |
| Quinolones | • Bone/tendon growth abnormality<br>• Avoid in pregnancy/children<br>• Rare QT prolongation |

## Urinary Tract Infection (UTI)

All UTIs present with dysuria, meaning:

- Frequency: urge to urinate often, without much urine coming out
- Urgency: "When you feel you have to go, do you feel you have to run to bathroom?"
- Burning

Frequency differs from polyuria; polyuria is an *increased volume* of urine. Polyuria is characteristic of diabetes. Frequency means that you go often but does not assume that much urine is made each time.

## Cystitis

Look for dysuria with:

- Suprapubic/bladder area pain
- Little or no fever
- UA >5–10 WBCs

In cystitis, you do not need to wait for the results of urine culture in order to start treatment.

### Treatment

- Nitrofurantoin 100 bid × 5 days
- Fosfomycin 3 g single dose
- TMP/SMZ DS 1 bid × 3 days

Extend the length of therapy for "complicated" cystitis. Men are treated longer. Men generally should not be getting UTIs unless there is an anatomic defect leading to the disorder. Women can easily have cystitis without an anatomic defect.

All men with UTI need renal/urinary imaging (U/S or CT).

Complications need 7 days of therapy. These are an obstruction or foreign body, such as:

- Stone
- Stricture
- Tumor, obstruction, neurogenic bladder
- Pregnancy
- Catheters
- Diabetes

## Pyelonephritis

Dysuria and UA with WBC and:

- Flank or "costovertebral angle" (CVA) tenderness and pain
- Fever
- Often much more ill-appearing patient than in cystitis
- UA often much higher WBC count than cystitis

Ultrasound or CT is needed to determine the cause of the UTI. If there is a stone, stricture, or obstruction, an imaging study is the only way to determine its presence. If there is an anatomic problem causing the pyelonephritis and it is not detected and repaired, there will be a recurrence.

In equivocal cases, confirm a diagnosis with sonogram or CT.

### Treatment

For outpatient care, give ciprofloxacin 750 bid for 10–14 days. Oral cipro at a higher dose (750 bid) has the same "area under curve" as IV cipro.

For inpatient care, any of the medications listed in the table (above) "Antibiotics for Gram-Negative Bacilli" is acceptable. Specific recommendations for pyelonephritis are:

- Ceftriaxone 1 g every 24 hours
- Ciprofloxacin
- Ampicillin and gentamicin
- Meropenem, beta-lactam/beta-lactamase combination (severe, complicated disease)

## Perinephric Abscess

A patient with pyelonephritis will not improve after 5–7 days of treatment. CT of the kidneys will show a collection under the capsule. CT-guided biopsy/aspiration is required. You cannot determine appropriate therapy without a culture, as therapy develops while the patient is on antibiotics.

**Perinephric abscess = resistant organism**

## Skin Infections

Skin infections are diagnosed by their appearance. Generally, there is no specific diagnostic test. Swab cultures are worse than useless and aspirations yield little. Bacteremia occurs in <5%.

Skin infections are an area of medicine that is impossible to learn from a book. You need to see them with an experienced person to know which ones are severe and which are mild.

## Presentation

**Cellulitis:**

- Deep in the subcutaneous tissues and dermis
- Drainage less common
- *Staphylococcus aureus* is most common organism
- Group A beta hemolytic *Streptococcus* (GAS) is less common (GAS used to be called *Streptococcus pyogenes.*)

**Erysipelas:**

- Bright red and warm to hot
- More superficial
- More often GAS
- Difficult to determine organism by appearance

**Impetigo:**

- Superficial
- Characterized by "weeping, crusting, and oozing" lesions that may be the color of honey

## Treatment

**Intravenous:**

- Oxacillin or nafcillin 1–2 g every 4 hours
- Cefazolin (Ancef) 1–2 g every 8 hours
- If no response after 2–3 days, switch to vancomycin
- If anaphylaxis to penicillin: vancomycin 1 g every 12 hours

Cefazolin is safe with when penicillin allergy presents as rash.

**Oral:**

- Dicloxacillin or cloxacillin 500 4x/day
- Cephalexin (Keflex) 500 4x/day
- MRSA
  - TMP/SMZ
  - Clindamycin

- Doxycycline
- Linezolid

**Topical:**

- Mupirocin (bactroban) or retapamulin

# Endocarditis

Look for fever and a new murmur or change in a murmur.

- Risks: injection drug use or prosthetic valves
- Rarely: embolic events (splinter hemorrhage, Roth spots in eye, Janeway/Osler's in hands and feet)
- Persistent bacteremia

## Diagnostic Tests

The first test to do is blood culture. Do 3 sets of cultures to excluded endocarditis. Sustained or persistent bacteremia is strong evidence of endocarditis.

If blood cultures are positive, get an echocardiogram.

- Transthoracic echo (TTE) first (60% sensitive, 95–99% specific)
- If TTE is negative and there is persistent bacteremia, do transesophageal echo (TEE) next (>95% sensitive, >95% specific)

Positive blood cultures + vegetation on echo = **endocarditis**

## Treatment

In those with strong suspicion of endocarditis, start treatment as soon as 3 blood cultures are obtained.

**Empiric therapy: vancomycin *and* gentamicin**

Once the blood cultures grow and the specific organism and sensitivity is known, switch antibiotics. Do not continue vancomycin for an organism that is sensitive to penicillin.

Specific therapies are as follows. The antibiotics do not have to be completed in hospital. Arrange for home antibiotics.

**Round Saver**

If an organism is sensitive, vancomycin is less effective than oxacillin in terms of killing bacteria.

| Specific Organism | Treatment | Duration |
|---|---|---|
| *Staphylococcus aureus:* sensitive | Oxacillin, nafcillin, or cefazolin | 6 weeks |
| *Staphylococcus aureus:* resistant | Vancomycin or daptomycin | 6 weeks |
| Viridans group strepto-coccus | Ceftriaxone, ampicillin, or penicillin | 4 weeks |
| Enterococcus: penicillin-sensitive | Both ampicillin and gentamicin | 6 weeks |

Add rifampin for prosthetic valve endocarditis.

To determine **who needs immediate surgery**, look for:

- Valve rupture:
  - Look for sudden dyspnea and rales
  - Do not wait! Surgery **cures** the endocarditis!
  - No amount of antibiotics will re-attach a ruptured valve!
- Abscess of heart
- Recurrent emboli while on antibiotics
- Fungal endocarditis

**Round Saver**

**You must read more** around cases you see!

- Prosthetic valves: It is very hard to cure an infected artificial valve

*S. bovis* really does require a colonoscopy.

## HIV/AIDS

There is little difference any longer in distinguishing between HIV and AIDS. On a Medicine rotation you will see only 2 groups of people admitted:

- Newly diagnosed or noncompliant patients with opportunistic infections
- Older patients admitted for other reasons in whom HIV is a chronic disease such as diabetes

Because the death rate from HIV is down by 80–90% compared to 20 years ago, patients are now commonly living into their 60s and 70s and admitted with the same medical conditions as anyone else, such as MI and stroke. For these patients, simply continue the HIV medications they routinely take. In those who are newly diagnosed or admitted for opportunistic infections from noncompliance with antiretroviral therapy (ART), begin treatment.

When patients are in the hospital, make sure to continue their HIV medications.

### Antiretroviral Therapy (ART)

The goal of therapy is undetectable viral load.

Normal CD4 count is 800–1,100/μL but there are virtually no opportunistic infections until $CD_4$ drops to nearly 200 cells. The recommended starting point for ART has changed many times over the last 15 years. $CD_4$ cells drop at a rate of 50–100 cells per year, so it will take 5–10 years for a person to drop from a normal level to one in which illness begins.

In addition, the average **increase** in $CD_4$ cells is 200–250/μL with the use of ART. There is concern about damage to the immune system during the wait until the $CD_4$ drops to <350, so therapy is best initiated when the count goes <500 to make sure the count stays well above that at which opportunistic infections occur.

Some experts would begin at any $CD_4$, even >500, but it must be remembered that:

- The recommended point of initiation has changed frequently.
- It takes years for a $CD_4$ to drop from 700/μL to 200, thus it is hard to prove a mortality benefit when starting at this high a count.
- Medications have adverse effects.
- Intermittent periods of noncompliance will create a resistant virus.

## Initiating ART: Clear Answers

- Keep $CD_4$ cells >350/μL to prevent opportunistic infections.
- Most everyone would start ART at <500 $CD_4$ cells.
- All pregnant women with HIV should be treated immediately with ART.
- Coinfection with hepatitis B or C needs ART to prevent liver damage.
- Start right away in **all** those with opportunistic infections.
- Start with the following:
    - At least 3 drugs from 2 different classes
    - 1x/day combination to make compliance easy
    - Tenofovir/emtricitabine with 1 of the following:
        - Nonnucleoside: efavirenz
        - Protease inhibitor: atazanavir

- Darunavir
- Raltegravir (an integrase inhibitor)
- All combinations are 3 meds 1x/day.

**Round Saver**

All protease inhibitors increase glucose and lipids.

Some physicians would start ART for every HIV-positive person.

**Boosting** is adding ritonavir to a protease inhibitor to increase its blood level and efficacy. Adding a small dose of ritonavir (100 mg/day) to most protease inhibitors markedly increases their levels without the extra toxicity of higher doses of ritonavir or the other medications.

**Adverse Effects of HIV Medications**

| Nucleoside Reverse Transcriptase | Adverse Effect |
|---|---|
| Zidovudine | Macrocytic anemia |
| Didanosine, stavudine | Pancreatitis, neuropathy |
| Tenofovir | Renal, RTA |
| Abacavir | Skin, Stevens-Johnson |
| Protease inhibitors (class effect) | Hyperlipidemia, hyperglycemia |
| Nonnucleoside: efavirenz | Teratogenicity |

Note that all nucleosides cause lactic acidosis.

## Viral Sensitivity Testing

Before starting therapy, genotyping should be done to be sure that even a treatment-naïve person has a virus that is fully sensitive to the medications that will be started.

- Genotype all treatment failures.
- Start at least 2 new drugs to which the organism is sensitive.
- Drop drugs to which there is resistance.

- Use viral-load testing to determine treatment success or failure.

### Post-Exposure Prophylaxis (PEP)

Any serious injury with a blood-containing sharp instrument from an HIV-positive patient must be treated with a combination of 3 drugs for 1 month.

- Risk of transmission with no PEP is 0.3% or 1/300.
- PEP medications decrease this by at least 80%.
- Extra written consent is not needed to HIV-test the source patient any longer.
  - Consent for HIV testing is needed, though it does not need to be in writing.
- PEP for needle sticks on HIV-unknown sources is generally NOT needed.
- Kissing, urine, and stool do not transmit HIV.

### Pregnancy

As soon as you learn that an HIV-positive person is pregnant, initiate treatment. If the patient is already on ART and well controlled (viral load undetectable), just continue treatment.

- Only efavirenz is teratogenic.
- C-section at delivery is only needed if viral load is >1,000 at delivery.
- **HIV-positive mothers must not breastfeed, ever; even if viral load is undetectable, no breastfeeding.**

When viral load is <20 (undetectable), perinatal transmission is <1%.

# HEAD AND NECK INFECTIONS

## Sinusitis

Most sinusitis is viral. The majority of cases resolve with no antibiotics because they are viral in etiology. Do not give antibiotics.

- Face pain, nasal congestion, and sometimes teeth pain
- Headache and fever
- Discolored nasal discharge
- Treat with acetaminophen and nasal steroids
  - Amoxicillin/clavulanic acid and decongestant (if fever and discolored discharge)

### Diagnostic Testing

The majority of those with sinusitis do not need radiologic testing. Do not culture the nasal discharge. Do not do nasal swabs.

If the diagnosis is unclear, do x-ray and either CT or MRI. For recurrent cases despite 3–4 rounds of empiric therapy, do a biopsy or nasal endoscopy for culture.

## Otitis Media

- Pain in ear
- Otoscopy with immobile, red, bulging tympanic membrane
- Empiric treatment with amoxicillin
- Azithromycin or clarithromycin with penicillin allergy
- If no response to amoxicillin in 2–3, days switch to amoxicillin-clavulanic acid or second-generation cephalosporin (loracarbef, cefdinir, ceftibuten, cefuroxime)

## Pharyngitis

The main issue is to identify patients who have Group A *Streptococcal* (GAS) pharyngitis. The remaining cases all resolve and are nonpathogenic. We want to identify those who need treatment without waiting for the results of throat culture. The "rapid antigen detection" test for GAS infection is extremely specific if positive, but at 80% sensitive is not great at excluding GAS infection. If suspicion is high, continue antibiotics with amoxicillin or penicillin while waiting for culture results. GAS pharyngitis is likely if there is:

- Pain on swallowing
- Fever by history
- Exudate on the pharynx/tonsils (it should scrape off)
- Cervical nodes
- Absence of cough (cough is lung infection, not pharynx)
- Absence of hoarseness (hoarseness if laryngitis—a virus)

The goal with pharyngitis is to identify and treat those at risk for glomerulonephritis or rheumatic fever.

## Lemiere's Syndrome

- Suppurative, septic thrombophlebitis of jugular vein and neurovascular bundle of neck
- Pain, swelling, tenderness, and redness along sternocleidomastoid
- Fever (>39°C), rigors, chills
- *Fusobacterium necrophorum*
- Blood cultures
- CT of neck
- Surgical debridement (emergency!)
- Unasyn, Zosyn, any carbapenem

## Influenza

Treat those with influenza in the first 48 hours after the onset of symptoms. Look for:

- Fever
- Arthralgia, myalgia, headache
- Fatigue, malaise
- Cough, sore throat

Diagnose with rapid antigen detection methods on nasopharyngeal wash if presentation is unclear.

Use oseltamivir or zanamivir in the first 48 hours of symptoms to shorten duration of illness.

## Lyme Disease

For an asymptomatic tick bite:

- Do not test or treat
- Tick needs 24–36 hours of attachment
- Must be an *Ixodes* tick

For rash:

- No serology needed
- Look for red ring with pale center
- Doxycycline, amoxicillin, or cefuroxime

For neurologic, cardiac, and joint manifestations:

- All need confirmation of Lyme with serology.
- Cranial nerve VII palsy and joint disease are treated with oral doxycycline or amoxicillin.
  - CN VII (facial) palsy is **not** CNS.
- CNS and cardiac disease are treated with IV ceftriaxone.

The most common cardiac lesion is AV block.

# SEXUALLY TRANSMITTED DISEASES

## Herpes Simplex

The vesicles of the genital area can be treated without testing.

- Acyclovir, valacyclovir, and famciclovir are equal in efficacy.
  - Acyclovir can cause renal insufficiency.
- Ulcers need confirmation with viral culture—grows in 2–3 days.

Treatment is oral; topical is worthless. For severe infection, use IV acyclovir 5 mg/kg every 8 hours. For acyclovir-resistant herpes simplex, use foscarnet.

## Syphilis

| Primary Syphilis | Secondary | Tertiary |
|---|---|---|
| Genital ulcer/chancre<br>Painless nodes | Skin rash, alopecia<br>Condylomata lata<br>Mucous patch | Neurological<br>Aortic rare |
| Darkfield most accurate<br>VDRL/RPR is 80% sensitive<br>FTA confirmatory | VDRL/RPR 99% sensitive<br>FTA confirms | CSF-FTA negative excludes<br>VDRL positive confirms |
| Single IM penicillin<br>Doxycycline for allergic | Single IM penicillin<br>Doxycycline for allergic | IV penicillin<br>Desensitize allergic |

Latent syphilis exists when the primary or secondary stage has resolved without treatment.

- Asymptomatic positive serology
- VDRL/RPR >1:8 and positive FTA

Treat with 3 IM shots of penicillin 1 week apart. In pregnancy, desensitize the penicillin-allergic patient.

**Round Saver**

Negative CSF-FTA is 99% sensitive.

With neurosyphilis, VDRL is positive in only 30–60% of patients. Use fluorescent treponemal antibody (FTA) in CSF to exclude neurosyphilis.

## Lymphogranuloma Venereum

- Painful matted, enlarged nodes
- Ulcer

Diagnose with chlamydia serology or aspiration. Treat with doxycycline.

## Urethritis

Urethritis is dysuria plus discharge.

- Urethral swab for Gram stain shows Gram-negative diplococci in men.
- Voided urine for nucleic acid amplification test (NAAT) for both gonococcus and chlamydia

Treat with ceftriaxone IM and azithromycin oral 1x. This is the same treatment for cervicitis.

## Cervicitis

- Dyspareunia and cervical discharge
- Self-administered vaginal swab for NAAT for gonorrhea and chlamydia

Treat with ceftriaxone IM and azithromycin oral 1x.

## Pelvic Inflammatory Disease (PID)

- Lower abdominal tenderness and lower abdominal pain in a woman
  - Don't forget the pregnancy test for all women with lower abdominal pain!!
- Cervical motion tenderness

If there is high fever and high WBC count, admit for IV antibiotics. Use cefoxitin (or cefotetan) and doxycycline.

## Noninfectious Causes of Fever

- Clots: deep vein thrombosis, pulmonary embolism
- Hematoma: any collection of blood can cause a fever
- Drugs
  - There is no test for drug fever. It can only be labeled as such once infectious causes are excluded.
- Postoperative
  - Major surgery is associated with fever.

**Fever of unknown origin (FUO)** is made only after initial testing is unrevealing. It is not an FUO when someone is admitted and the tests have not yet been done.

**Is there an identifiable cause or symptom?**

- Cough? Get x-ray and sputum culture.
- Dysuria? Get UA and possibly urethral swab or voided urine for NAAT for chlamydia/gonorrhea.
- Skin?
- Joint pain? Aspirate swollen joint for cell count >50,000.

**No identifiable source?** Obtain:

- Blood cultures, 2 sets drawn at 2 sites
- UA
- CXR

**Are blood, urine, and chest x-ray unrevealing, and fever persists?** This is now an FUO! Get one of the following:

- Abdominal/pelvic CT
  - CT usually done first for FUO because it is easy to do.
- Bone marrow biopsy
- Gallium scan

Also consult an infectious disease specialist.

# Nephrology 6

## ACUTE RENAL FAILURE

There is nothing in the physical exam that can tell you the etiology of acute renal failure. Nephrology is a laboratory-based specialty.

- Repeat all abnormal labs to confirm accuracy.
    - Multiple levels are essential to establish the trend: Improving? Worsening? Stable?
- Urinalysis (UA) and renal ultrasound (U/S) are essential for everyone with renal injury.

Renal failure is an emergency in the following scenarios:

- Hyperkalemia
- Metabolic acidosis
- Pericarditis
- Fluid overload
- Encephalopathy/altered mental status

**Round Saver**

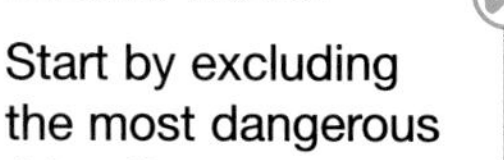

Start by excluding the most dangerous thing first.

When any of these conditions are present, you need to do the following:

- Make sure your resident/attending is informed.
- Arrange for dialysis.
- Get an EKG for hyperkalemia.

## Etiology

Blood urea nitrogen (BUN) to creatinine ratio is first in determining etiology.

**BUN/creatinine ratio:**

Ratio >20 to 1: pre-renal azotemia; decreased renal perfusion

Ratio 10 to 1: intra-renal (a problem inside the kidney)

## Diagnostic Testing

With suspected renal failure, the following tests should be done:

- BUN and creatinine
  - *Always* repeat them; never make a decision based on 1 lab value.
- Urinalysis, serum chemistry (potassium, sodium, bicarbonate)
- Renal ultrasound
- Urine osmolarity, urine sodium, protein:creatinine ratio (some patients only)

With acute renal failure, a 24-hour urine protein is useless.

On urinalysis, rhabdomyolysis would show with dip + for blood, without RBC.

**Round Saver** 

You will look foolish if you make big decisions on 1 abnormal test.

## Pre-Renal Azotemia

"Pre-renal" illness means the patient is having renal insufficiency from abnormal perfusion of the kidney. The kidney itself is normal and would function normally if transplanted into another person.

BUN:creatinine ratio 20:1 indicates pre-renal azotemia. Pre-renal azotemia is caused by:

- Dehydration/hypovolemia
- Hypotension of any kind
- CHF, especially after use of furosemide and diuretics
  - CHF causes edema but the kidneys are dry (underperfused)
- Hypoalbuminemia
- Renal artery stenosis
  - Affects the kidney like pre-renal azotemia (hypoperfusion) despite hypertension

### Diagnostic Testing

- **BUN:creatinine ratio at least >15:1** (often >20:1)
- Urine **sodium low** (**<20** mEq/L)
- Urine **osmolarity high** (**>500** mOsm)
- Fractional excretion of **sodium (FeNa) low** (<1%)
  - However, this adds nothing to simple low sodium
- Renal U/S:
  - Normal with acute disease
  - Shows small kidneys with chronic disease

> **Round Saver**
>
> Anyone who tortures you with learning FeNa calculations is wasting your time.

Treatment involves correcting the cause of the pre-renal azotemia and hydration.

# Acute Tubular Necrosis (ATN)

Acute tubular necrosis (ATN) is damage of the renal tubule (intrinsic renal injury), most often from a toxin. It is frequently accompanied by hypoperfusion of the kidney. ATN is caused by:

- Contrast material
- Drugs as toxins:
  - Aminoglycosides
  - Acyclovir
  - TMP/SMZ (i.e., Bactrim)
  - Amphotericin
  - Cisplatin
- Hypercalcemia
- Rhabdomyolysis/myoglobin
- Hemolysis/hemoglobin
- Allergic (acute) interstitial nephritis
- Crystals (uric acid, oxalate)

Chronic use of NSAIDs is a very common cause—perhaps the most common cause—of ATN.

## Diagnostic Testing

- BUN:creatinine ratio at least <**15:1 (often <10:1)**
- **Urine sodium high** (**>40** mEq/L)
- Urine **osmolarity low** (**<350** mOsm)
  - Fractional excretion of **sodium (FeNa) low (>1%)** (but this adds nothing to simple high sodium)
- Renal ultrasound: with acute disease, U/S is normal; with chronic disease, U/S shows small kidneys

### Treatment

There is no medication to reverse ATN. Treatment is based on stopping exposure to the toxin and preventing further damage. Once injury has occurred, you can only support the patient and wait to see if recovery occurs or, in severe injury, if dialysis is needed.

- Correct underlying cause
- Hydration in most cases

Loop diuretics such as furosemide are ineffective and even dangerous in ATN.

There is no treatment with contrast agents to reverse injury to the kidneys, so management is to prevent injury.

- Half-normal or normal (isotonic) saline: 1–2 liters before the procedure and 6 hours after
- N-acetylcysteine likely helps
- Sodium bicarbonate may help

Hydration is not given to every person getting contrast agents; it is given to those who have underlying renal dysfunction with an elevated creatinine (diabetics, those with hypertension, the elderly).

## Obstructive Uropathy (Post-Renal Failure)

Confirm the diagnosis:

- Is there a palpable bladder on exam?
  - You may feel it bulging above the pubic symphysis.
- Ultrasound:
  - Look for hydronephrosis; must be bilateral to cause renal failure
  - Ultrasound finds stones and cause of obstruction
- Placement of Foley (urinary catheter)
  - Bladder obstruction (e.g., BPH) will cause rapid production of high volumes of urine.

Note that the Foley catheter is uncomfortable. Do not place it unless truly required.

### Treatment

- Correct the underlying cause:
  - Prostate disease (benign hypertrophy, cancer)
  - Bladder or cervical cancer
  - Neurogenic bladder (multiple sclerosis, diabetes)
  - Stones (bladder)
  - Bilateral ureteral or urethral strictures
- Hydration
  - After obstruction is relieved there can be a marked diuresis. All the fluid that did not leave because of obstruction may now "flood" out of the body. Make sure to replace the fluid that was lost.

## Rhabdomyolysis

Look for:

- Sudden, severe muscular injury
- Seizures
- Trauma
- Extreme physical exercise/weight lifting

> **How NOT to Kill Your Patient**
>
> Watch for hyperkalemia and changes in EKG. A person can die from hyperkalemia. Start normal saline at high volume, e.g., 200–300 mL per hour, as it may take 3–4 days for the increased creatine phosphokinase (CPK) to clear.

### Diagnostic Testing

- Urine dipstick shows a dipstick positive for blood and hemoglobin.
- No red cells are seen.
- Urine myoglobin is most specific, but never available immediately.
- CPK level must be elevated to 20,000–50,000 to be considered significant.
- Calcium can be low; damaged muscle "sucks up" calcium.

A massive release of hemoglobin is managed in the same way as rhabdomyolysis.

## Allergic (Acute) Interstitial Nephritis (AIN)

Look for ATN and the recent start of a new drug. Fever plus rash is highly suggestive. Rash, hemolysis, and AIN are all caused by same drugs.

The drugs most frequently associated with AIN are:

- Penicillin, sulfa, allopurinol, phenytoin
- Rifampin
- PPIs
- Ciprofloxacin
- Lamotrigine

### Diagnostic Testing

- Rising BUN and creatinine in 10:1 ratio with normal renal ultrasound
- Urinalysis: WBCs
- Eosinophils on urine by Hansel's or Wright stain
    - Urinalysis cannot identify that the WBCs are eosinophils.
- CBC with eosinophilia is HIGHLY suggestive of AIN if present, but means nothing if CBC is normal.

Treatment is to stop the drugs and wait for resolution. Consider steroids (prednisone, methylprednisolone) if the creatinine continues to rise. Steroids for AIN are not proven, but use if there are no other options.

## Crystals: Uric Acid and Oxalate

Etiology:

- Uric acid
  - Look for gout or tumor lysis after chemotherapy
  - Fluids
  - Allopurinol or febuxostat
  - Pegloticase or rasburicase

Don't start allopurinol during an acute flare of gout.

- Oxalate
  - Look for ethylene glycol (antifreeze) overdose.
  - "Envelope-shaped" crystals on UA
  - Treatment: fomepizole

## Chronic Use of NSAIDs

NSAIDs can damage the kidney by:

- Direct toxin
- Allergic interstitial nephritis
- Nephrotic syndrome
- Vascular insufficiency
- Papillary necrosis

## Papillary Necrosis

- Sudden onset flank pain after NSAID use in a person with chronic kidney disease
- Patient often passes "necrotic kidney pieces" in urine
- Diagnose with CT scan: "bumpy" appearance of inner kidney
- No specific treatment

## Hypercalcemia

1. Give large volumes of normal saline: 1–2 liters in first hour.
2. Calcitonin works fast! *Make sure it was actually given*, not just ordered.
3. Zoledronic acid or pamidronate (bisphosphonates) take a few days to work.

Remember that hypercalcemia leads to nephrogenic diabetes insipidus and thus massive free water loss, which can be 5–10 liters.

Look for:

- Nausea, vomiting, constipation, and abdominal pain
- Confusion or altered mental status
- History of cancer (hypercalcemia of malignancy)

**Round Saver**

Check the medication administration record first! Be 100% sure the medication ordered *was actually given*.

For more on hypercalcemia, see Chapter 2: Endocrinology.

# Dialysis

Dialysis needs to be done when the patient is developing life-threatening complications/manifestations of renal failure.

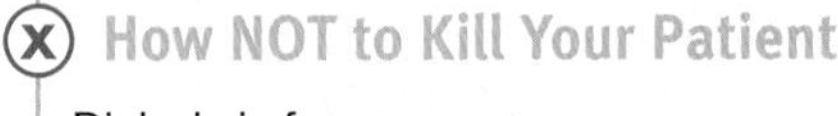


Dialysis is for:

- Severe acidosis
- Pericarditis
- Encephalopathy/confusion
- Fluid overload
- Hyperkalemia

When these conditions are present, make sure the nephrologist has been called so dialysis can be arranged for **that day**. If it is Friday night, these manifestations cannot wait until Monday for dialysis.

The indication for dialysis is not a specific level of BUN or creatinine. These manifestations occur exclusively below a creatinine clearance of 30 mL/min, usually <10 mL/min.

The key to rapid and efficient dialysis is **vascular access**.

- Emergent = central venous line
- Chronic = fistula/AV graft

## Chronic Manifestations of End-Stage Renal Failure

| Manifestation | Treatment |
|---|---|
| Anemia | Erythropoietin |
| Hypocalcemia | Vitamin D replacement |
| Hyperphosphatemia | • Calcium acetate/phosphate<br>• Lanthanum<br>• Sevelamer |
| Bone (osteomalacia) | • Vitamin D<br>• Calcium |
| Hypertension | Often requires 3–4 medications |
| Hypermagnesemia | Restricted magnesium in diet |

# HYPERTENSION

## Hypertensive Crisis

Hypertensive crisis is defined as **acute symptoms of end-organ damage plus severe hypertension**. There is no single blood pressure level at which to define a hypertensive crisis. If there are no symptoms, there is no "crisis." This is very important.

Blood pressure levels >160/100 mmHg or >180/120 mmHg can be very frightening to caregivers. By themselves, however, high blood pressure levels are not considered a hypertensive crisis.

Look for:

- Confusion
- Chest pain
- Visual disturbance with headache
- Dyspnea
- Decreased urinary output

### Treatment

- Labetalol, enalaprilat, hydralazine, or any other IV medication
- Do not reduce blood pressure >25% in the first few hours or you may precipitate a stroke

Round Saver 

Some attendings will call hypertensive crisis an "emergency," "acceleration," or "urgency." Don't disagree! The name doesn't matter.

## Hypertension

Do not label anyone as being hypertensive based on a single elevated blood pressure reading. This is especially true of those admitted to the hospital for acute illness. (You might be hypertensive, too, if you were taken to a strange new place where you felt you had lost all control to the care of strangers just when you were weak and vulnerable.)

Make sure you do **not** label as "hypertensive" someone with:

- Pain
- Anxiety
- Alcohol withdrawal
- Psychiatric disturbance

### Treatment

#### Inpatient Care of Hypertension

Although the standard of care for initial management of hypertension has long been thiazides, in the hospital you should focus on the other medical problems the patient may have. Expect the majority of patients to come in with an additional medical problem. With newly diagnosed hypertension, your goal is to ensure that the patient is given a blood pressure medication that will treat both the hypertension as well as the other existing problem.

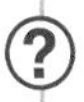

## Things You Will Be Asked on Rounds

- Whether patient is usually on antihypertensive medications; if so, restart those
  - Were doses checked to make sure the correct regular dose was started?
- If private/ambulatory care doctor was called
  - Make sure you know if the blood pressure problem is old or new

Do not label a condition as "uncontrolled hypertension" when it is a case of simple failure to restart the patient's regular medications or correct the dose. People miss things. Trust no one.

### Round Saver

You *will* catch mistakes if you look. Put the patient's needs above your grade.

With hypertension that has compelling indications, the "compelling indications" are the same for both hospitalized and ambulatory outpatients. However, anyone who has been hospitalized as an inpatient is far more likely to have hypertension *plus* another medical problem. For this reason, treatment is more important in the inpatient setting.

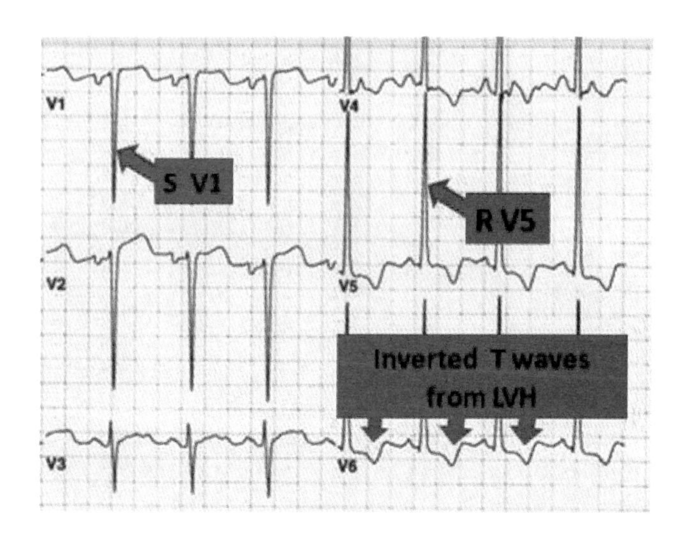


**Deep S-wave V1 + tall R-wave V5 >35 mm = LVH.**
**LVH causes T-wave inversion and ST abnormalities, which make interpretation for ischemia nearly impossible.**

| Compelling Indication | Class of Medication |
|---|---|
| Coronary disease (CAD) | Beta blockers (metoprolol) |
| CHF | • Beta blockers (metoprolol, carvedilol)<br>• ACE inhibitors (any in class)<br>• ARB (if intolerant of ACE inhibitors)<br>• Aldosterone antagonists (spironolactone)<br>• Hydralazine/nitrates if hyp**er**kalemia |
| Diabetes | ACE inhibitors or ARBs |
| Asthma/COPD | Avoid beta blockers, but TRY THEM if there is coronary disease too! |
| Depression | Avoid beta blockers |
| Renal insufficiency | ACE inhibitors protect kidneys |

There are some **common errors in hypertension management**. For instance, several treatments formerly thought to be dangerous or contraindicated are indeed acceptable to use. One example is the mortality benefit of metoprolol in CAD; it is more important than adverse effects such as claudication.

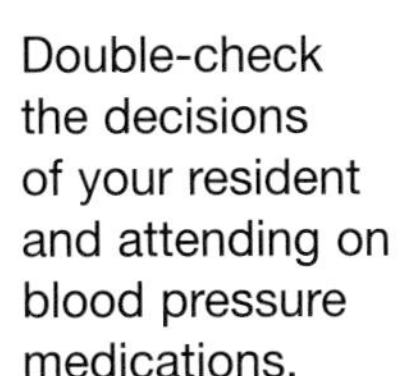


- PAD and CAD: metoprolol should be used
- COPD and CAD: metoprolol can be tolerated in 70–80% of patients
- Diabetes and renal insufficiency: ACE inhibitors and ARBs **protect** the kidney. Use them to keep the patient off dialysis
    - Using ACE inhibitors and ARBs does not absolve you of the need to monitor BUN, creatinine, and potassium.
- In the absence of compelling indications, beta blockers, calcium channel blockers, ACE inhibitors, and ARBs are all okay to use.

Metoprolol is safer in COPD and PAD than initially thought.

## Ambulatory Care of Hypertension

- Repeat the blood pressure several times over several days to weeks. There is no hurry in the absence of symptoms.
- Hypertension is defined as >140/90 mmHg. No one knows what to do about "pre-hypertension." Everyone should exercise, eat right, and lose weight.
- Hypertension in diabetes or renal insufficiency is >130/80 mmHg.
- Lifestyle modifications
    - Weight loss is the most effective lifestyle modification. It is also the only one that can be measured.
    - Lifestyle modifications should be tried for 3–6 months in motivated, stable patients.

- Medications
  - If there are no compelling indications as listed above, start with a thiazide.
  - If there are any of the compelling indications listed above (CHF, CAD, DM), **do not** start a thiazide. Instead, use the drug associated with the compelling indication.
- For severe hypertension, use a thiazide plus CCB, ACE inhibitor, or beta blocker
  - If blood pressure >160/100 mmHg, 2 medications must be started. One alone isn't sufficient.

# ELECTROLYTE DISORDERS

## Potassium (K) Disorders

Potassium (K) abnormalities are extremely common in the hospital. Whether the level is up or down, potassium causes:

- Arrhythmias that can easily be fatal
- Muscle weakness
- Nephrogenic diabetes insipidus with low potassium

**Round Saver**

Potassium disorders are a "must read" subject.

In all cases of potassium abnormality, always recheck the level after you have treated it. Do not wait until the next day to recheck potassium abnormality.

**How NOT to Kill Your Patient**

If potassium is >6.0 mEq/L, stop reading this book and call your PGY1 resident immediately. High levels of potassium (>6.5 mEq/L) need:

- EKG immediately
- Repeat the level
- Kayexalate orally (30–60 g) or by enema
- Possibly insulin (10 units) and dextrose (25 g or 1 ampule)
- Bicarbonate if the hyperkalemia is from metabolic acidosis (pH <7.2)
- Possibly albuterol
- Continuous cardiac monitoring (e.g., telemetry)

## Hyperkalemia

When EKG abnormalities exist in the presence of hyperkalemia, tests will show peaked T-waves or wide QRS.

- Give immediate calcium chloride (1 g) or calcium gluconate intravenously
- Make sure the Kayexalate and insulin/dextrose ordered was actually given

The causes of hyperkalemia are:

- Renal failure/insufficiency
- Medications
  - ACE inhibitors/ARBs
  - Aldosterone antagonists (spironolactone, eplerenone)
  - Beta blockers
- Acidosis (metabolic more common)
- Diabetes, especially DKA
- Cell breakdown
  - Tumor lysis
  - Rhabdomyolysis
  - Hemolysis
- Adrenal insufficiency/Addison's disease

> **Round Saver** 
>
> Hyperkalemia with changes in EKG means run, don't walk!

## Hypokalemia

Low potassium causes cardiac and muscular problems as well.

- Maximum dose is 10 mEq/hr **intravenously** on regular hospital floor.
- In intensive care, 20–30 mEq/hr can be given with continuous cardiac monitor.
- There is no maximum dose on oral replacement.
- Usual dose is **4–5 mEq/kg per point** of total body potassium. Do not give it all in 1 dose.

- 10 mEq KCl IV raises blood level by 0.1 mEq/L
- If you replace lots of potassium but the level does not go up, check the magnesium level. Low magnesium will cause urinary leakage of potassium, thereby preventing potassium correction.

With hypokalemia, the EKG will show "U" waves, an extra wave after the T-wave.

The causes of hypokalemia are:

- Urine loss: loop diuretics
- Low magnesium
- Metabolic alkalosis from transcellular shift of potassium into cells
- High aldosterone states
  - Conn's syndrome (primary hyperaldosteronism)
  - Cushing's syndrome
  - Prednisone use
  - Licorice (real black licorice contains aldosterone)
  - Bartter's syndrome (salt loss from loop of Henle)
- Beta-agonist overdose (albuterol)

Potassium causes cardiac problems, not CNS disturbance.

## Sodium Disorders

All sodium disorders, whether from high or low sodium, cause neurologic abnormalities when severe. Look for:

- Lethargy
- Confusion
- Altered mental status
- Seizures and coma (severe cases)

Sodium causes CNS problems, not rhythm disturbance.

## Hyponatremia

Normal sodium level is 135–145 mEq/L. However, mild hyponatremia with levels of 130–134 mEq/L are common, with no symptoms or the need for treatment.

The key to sodium disorder management is not the numerical sodium level, but rather the accompanying symptoms. Even if sodium 125–130 mEq/L, there is often no required treatment and only fluid restriction.

Treatment is based on etiology. The first step in assessing etiology is the fluid status of the patient. Is there fluid overload? dehydration? Is the volume status normal?

**Etiology of Hyponatremia by Fluid Status**

| Normal | Overload | Volume Depletion |
| --- | --- | --- |
| • SIADH<br>• Psychogenic polydipsia<br>• Hypothyroidism<br>• Addison's<br>• Hyperglycemia | • CHF<br>• Cirrhosis<br>• Nephrotic syndrome | • Addison's (adrenal)<br>• These **only** cause low sodium with free water replacement:<br>  ◦ GI, skin, urine loss |

For every 100 mg/dL above normal of glucose, there is an artificial drop of sodium or 1.6 mEq. This is a type of pseudohyponatremia. Treatment is correction of the glucose level.

Remember: glucose up 100 means sodium down 1.6.

## Syndrome of Inappropriate ADH (SIADH)

Patients with SIADH are neither edematous nor volume-overloaded. Symptoms are similar to other sodium disorders.

- Entirely related to severity of level of sodium
- CNS

Mild disease with sodium 125–134 mEq/L generally has no symptoms. If sodium level drops very slowly, the person can develop a profoundly low sodium level without any symptoms. A slowly dropping sodium level can reach a level of 115 or 120 mEq/L without presentation of symptoms.

SIADH has the following causes:

- CNS disease of any type: tumor, trauma, subdural hematoma, meningitis, encephalitis
- Lung disease of any type: pneumonia, TB, PE, atelectasis, any form of cancer
- Neoplasia
- Medications: carbamazepine, SSRIs, vincristine

SIADH leads to hyponatremia because there is inappropriately concentrated urine despite a low blood level of sodium. The urine sodium concentration is also inappropriately high despite a low blood level of sodium.

A normal person with low serum sodium should make a **maximally dilute** urine with an osmolarity of 50–100 mOsm and a urine sodium that is maximally low at <10 mEq/L. In SIADH, both the urine osmolarity and urine sodium are higher than they should be.

| | Normal | SIADH |
|---|---|---|
| **Urine osmolarity** | <100 mOsm | >Serum osmolarity<br>(though >100 mOsm is likely SIADH) |
| **Urine sodium** | <10 mEq | >20 mEq |

Treatment of SIADH depends on the severity of illness.

- Mild disease (no symptoms): fluid restriction
- Moderate disease (moderate confusion): saline and loop diuretic
- Severe disease (seizure, coma, profound confusion): hypertonic (3%) saline; conivaptan/tolvaptan
- Chronic disease: tolvaptan or demeclocycline

It is important to note the rate of correction.

1. Go slow, either up or down.
2. Do **not** correct sodium by more than 0.5–1 point per hour in asymptomatic or mildly symptomatic persons. Asymptomatic persons do not need faster correction than 12 points per 24 hours.
3. Severe illness (seizures/coma) can be corrected at 1–2 mEq/per hour
   - Rapid rise in sodium leads to central pontine myelinolysis.
   - Rapid drop in sodium leads to cerebral edema and seizures.
4. Normal saline alone, without a diuretic, can worsen SIADH. Saline has an osmolarity of 308. Urine in SIADH can have an osmolarity of ≥500–1,000. If you give saline in SIADH, you will drive the serum sodium down even further. You must use a loop diuretic with saline to get rid of the extra free water.

**How NOT to Kill Your Patient**

With SIADH, **do not use saline alone.**

## Hypernatremia

High sodium levels make patients confused and encephalopathic. Treatment of hypernatremia is easier because the initial therapy is always to hydrate the patient. At the beginning, any type of fluid will correct the sodium because the sodium level of saline is only 154 mEq/L.

1. Give 1–2 liters of saline in the first hour.
2. Ask your resident about switching to D5W or half-normal saline after the first few liters of saline.
3. Recheck the serum sodium frequently since no matter what fluid you choose, the answer is always: HYDRATE and REPEAT the chemistries in 1–2 hours for severe disease.
4. Calculating free water loss helps because we often markedly underestimate how much volume the patient is really missing.

For example, a 100 kg man with a sodium of only 160 (20 above normal) is missing 9 liters of fluid.

Remember:

- **Hypotensive = normal saline**
- **Normal volume = half normal**

### Etiology of Hypernatremia

Free water loss:

- Skin: sweating, burns, skin loss
- Urine: diuretics without free water replacement
- GI: diarrhea without free water replacement
- Diabetes insipidus
  - Central: head trauma, hypoxia, infection, tumor, granulomatous disease
  - Nephrogenic: low potassium, high calcium, sickle cell disease or trait

The only etiology that is really critical to acute management is **diabetes insipidus (DI)**. If DI exists, you cannot correct the disorder unless ADH (vasopressin) is given.

| Diagnosis of DI | | |
|---|---|---|
| **Disease** | **Dehydration (Skin/Urine Loss)** | **Diabetes Insipidus** |
| Urine volume | **Decreased** | **Increased** |
| Urine sodium | Low | Low |
| Urine osmolarity | **High** | **Low** |

To distinguish central DI from nephrogenic DI, do not be afraid to measure the urine osmolarity before and after giving ADH (vasopressin). You should not consider this a dangerous or complicated test.

- Central DI: urine osmolarity **rises** after vasopressin
- Nephrogenic DI: urine osmolarity **does not change** after vasopressin

To treat central DI, replace ADH as DDAVP (vasopressin). To treat nephrogenic DI, correct the underlying cause (potassium, calcium). Give thiazides or NSAIDs if there is no identifiable cause.

Repeat the sodium level frequently. Use the right fluids to make sure you go in the right direction.

# Acid-Base Disturbances

Normal values are as follows:

| | Normal | Range | High | Low |
|---|---|---|---|---|
| pH | 7.40 | 7.36–7.44 | Alkalosis | Acidosis |
| $pCO_2$ | 40 | 36–44 | Respiratory acidosis | Respiratory alkalosis |
| $HCO_3^-$ | 24 | 22–26 | Metabolic alkalosis | Metabolic acidosis |

The first step in any acid-base disturbance is to ask:

- What is the pH of the ABG?
- Does the bicarbonate match it? (acidosis vs. alkalosis)
- Does the $pCO_2$ match it? (acidosis vs. alkalosis)

## Arterial Blood Gas (ABG) Evaluation

| Acidosis (pH <7.36) | |
|---|---|
| **Primary disturbance is...** | |
| $HCO_3^-$ Low | $pCO_2$ High |
| Metabolic acidosis | Respiratory acidosis |
| Sepsis/lactate<br>Hypotension<br>Hypoperfusion<br>DKA<br>Uremia<br>Methanol | COPD<br>Respiratory failure<br>Opiate overdose |

| Alkalosis (pH >7.44) | |
|---|---|
| **Primary disturbance is...** | |
| $HCO_3^-$ High | $pCO_2$ High |
| Metabolic alkalosis | Respiratory alkalosis |
| Volume loss<br>Conn's<br>Cushing<br>Increased aldosterone | Hyperventilation of any kind<br>Pain<br>Anxiety<br>Fever<br>Anemia |

Note the following important relationships.

- Every time serum bicarbonate is newly down, **do ABG**.
- For every $pCO_2$ change of 10, pH should change by 0.08.
- Metabolic acidosis should be compensated by respiratory alkalosis.
- Metabolic disturbances get *immediate* respiratory compensation.
- Acute respiratory problems need 24–36 hours for full metabolic compensation.

New changes in serum bicarbonate need urgent ABG to investigate.

## Nephrolithiasis

Look for:

- Sudden, overwhelming, severe flank pain
- Radiation to groin
- Hematuria
- No tenderness on physical
- No fever

**Fever and tenderness = pyelonephritis**

### Management

1. Pain medication is **more** important than waiting for the ultrasound!
2. Ketorolac (toradol) is #1 drug for renal colic, but getting the patient out of pain is the **most** important thing no matter what you use!
3. Hydration, UA, renal U/S or renal CT is good to do, but pain medications are more important!

Make sure there is no obstruction after the pain is relieved.

### Treatment

For long-term management:

- Small stones <5 mm will pass spontaneously in >90%.
- Stones 5–8 mm may pass with help from nifedipine and tamsulosin (Flomax).
- Stones >5–8 mm need lithotripsy or surgical removal.
- Oversecretors of calcium may need thiazides to take calcium out of the urine. Restricting calcium in diet only increases oxalate absorption.

Do not restrict calcium in the diet.

## Renal Tubular Acidosis (RTA)

Look for:

- Metabolic acidosis with normal anion gap
- Hyperchloremic
- Urine pH is key to the diagnosis!

The body is acidotic on the basis of a renal tubular problem. Urine can be either acid (pH <5.4) or alkaline (pH >5.5).

Anion gap = sodium ($Na^+$) – ($HCO_3^-$ + $Cl^-$)
Normal anion gap: 6–12

Normal anion gap with metabolic acidosis = RTA or diarrhea.

| Types of RTA | | |
|---|---|---|
| | **Proximal** | **Distal** |
| Defect | Can't absorb $HCO_3^-$ | Can't excrete $H^+$ |
| Urine pH | Briefly high, then low | High (>5.5) |
| Stones | Urine pH low, no stone | pH high = stones |
| Test | Bicarb given, urinary pH rises | Acid given, urinary pH stays high |
| Treatment | Diuretics give volume contraction alkalosis | High-dose bicarbonate replacement |

Hyporeninemic hypoaldosteronism (type IV RTA) is characterized as follows:

- Diabetic with normal anion gap metabolic acidosis
- Hyperkalemia
- Hyperchloremia (which is why anion gap is normal)
- Continued high urine sodium on a salt-restricted diet
- Treat with fludrocortisone

## Polycystic Kidney Disease

- Causes recurrent kidney stones and pyelonephritis
- Leads to end-stage renal disease
- Subarachnoid hemorrhage is rare (<5%)
- U/S or CT is most accurate
- Cysts occur in multiple places in body (liver, ovary)
- Mitral valve prolapse and diverticulosis
- No specific therapy: treat stones and infection as they arise

# GLOMERULAR DISEASES

## Glomerulonephritis

All forms of glomerulonephritis can cause:

- Hematuria (look for "dysmorphic RBCs")
- Proteinuria
- Red cell casts
- Occasionally be "rapidly progressive"
- Very severe ones lead to nephrotic syndrome

### Diagnostic Testing

For all cases, do the following tests:

- Urinalysis
- Protein:creatinine ratio
- Renal U/S
- Some need a renal biopsy
  - Idiopathic nephrotic syndrome
  - IgA nephropathy
  - SLE nephritis to establish treatment

## IgA Nephropathy

- Most common cause of acute glomerulonephritis in United States
- No characteristic systemic manifestations or blood tests
- IgA levels are not reliable
- No treatment proven to reverse it
- When renal function and proteinuria worsen, use
  - Prednisone
  - ACE inhibitors
  - Fish oil
- Many end up on dialysis or needing a transplant

## Henoch-Schonlein Purpura (HSP)

HSP presents with:

- GI symptoms: abdominal pain, diarrhea
- Joint pain
- Skin lesions: purpura (non-blanching) purple lesions of lower extremities
- Renal insufficiency or hematuria/proteinuria
- Vast majority (>95%) resolve spontaneously!
- Small percentage who progress get treated like IgA nephropathy since HSP is an idiopathic IgA disorder

## SLE Nephritis

Kidney biopsy is the only way to establish severity.

  - Sclerosis: no therapy
  - Nonproliferative: steroids alone
  - Proliferative: steroids and either cyclophosphamide or mycophenolate

## Post-Streptococcal Glomerulonephritis (PSGN)

- Hypertension, dark urine, periorbital edema
- 1–2 weeks after streptococcal infection of **either** skin or pharynx
- Blood tests
  - Antistreptolysin O (ASLO) titer
  - Anti-DNAse
  - Antihyaluronidase
- Culture throat for streptococcus
- Treat with
  - Amoxicillin (even though does not clearly help, use it!)
  - Control hypertension
  - Diuretics sometimes
  - Vast majority recover

Biopsy is rarely needed for PSGN or Henoch-Schonlein.

## Wegener's Granulomatosis

Wegener's is a systemic vasculitis. It predominantly affects the upper respiratory tract (otitis, sinusitis), lung, and kidney.

- Also affects:
  - Joint pain and skin lesions
  - Eye (uveitis, iritis)
  - Neurological (mononeuritis multiplex, stroke in young person)
  - GI pain and bleeding
- C-ANCA
- Biopsy is indispensible
- Treat with steroids and cyclophosphamide

## Polyarteritis Nodosa

- No lung/respiratory manifestations
- History of hepatitis B or C
- GI problem most prominent
- P-ANCA in 20%
- GI angiogram or sural nerve biopsy

Other manifestations and treatment are the same as Wegener's.

## Churg-Strauss Syndrome

Churg-Strauss presents like Wegener's but without upper respiratory problems.

- Asthma and eosinophilia prominent
- P-ANCA best initial test
- Biopsy and treat like Wegener's

### Microscopic Polyangiitis

Microscopic polyangiitis also presents like Wegener's but without otitis/sinusitis.

- Use P-ANCA, not C-ANCA
- No granulomas on biopsy

## Nephrotic Syndrome

Any of the glomerular diseases can cause nephrotic syndrome. Nephrotic syndrome is a measure of severity of disease, not a specific etiology. If the damage is sufficient to the kidney that there is >3.5 grams of protein lost per day then the blood level will drop and edema will develop. Hyperlipidemia develops because there is a loss of the lipoproteins on the surface of VLDLs and LDLs that allow their clearance from the bloodstream.

Nephrotic syndrome is defined as:

- Hyp**ER**protein**URIA** >3.5 grams/24 hours
- Hyp**O**protein**EMIA**
- Edema
- Hyperlipidemia

Other manifestations of nephrotic syndrome are clotting (thrombophilia from urinary loss of protein C, protein S, and antithrombin), and iron deficiency from urine loss of transferrin.

### Diagnostic Testing

- UA: massive proteinuria >4+
- Protein-to-creatinine ratio >3.5:1
- Hyperlipidemia

A protein:creatinine ratio is just as accurate as 24-hour urine test. (24-hour urine is not needed and harder to do.)

Renal biopsy is the most accurate test. There are several causes of nephrotic syndrome that can be diagnosed only from renal biopsy. They have no specific blood test and no specific physical finding. Examples are:

- Minimal change disease
- Membranous
- Focal segmental
- Mesangial
- Membranoproliferative

Since none of these has a specific physical finding or a specific blood test, the only way to confirm their presence is to do the renal biopsy. Patients may simply choose to be treated with steroids (prednisone) for 12 weeks and then undergo biopsy if there is no response.

Treatment is oral steroids (prednisone) for 12 weeks. Add cyclophosphamide if there is no response.

**Round Saver**

Remember, your first duty is to the patient.

# Neurology 7

## Stroke

Stroke, also called "cerebrovascular accident" or CVA, is most often caused by an embolus coming from the heart, resulting in the sudden onset of neurological deficit. It is nonhemorrhagic in 80–85% and hemorrhagic in 15–20%. It is absolutely contraindicated to give any antiplatelet therapy until after the CT is done!

> **Round Saver**
> Think of CVA as CAD of the brain.

Because CVA often leads to speech deficit, you should expect to take history from family, friends, and caregivers. Precise details of timing may not be possible if the person woke up with the defect. When a person wakes with symptoms, timing is automatically assumed to be longer than 4.5 hours and outside the range for thrombolytic therapy (e.g., tPA).

### What to Ask About

- "When did symptoms start?"
- "Have they been getting better or worse?"
- "Do you have a headache?" (sign of a possible bleed)
- "Do you have difficulty swallowing?"
- "Did you lose consciousness?"
- "Do you feel unsteady when you stand?"
- "Are you having difficulty urinating, or are you losing your urine?" (incontinence)

Many patients have a history of:

- Hypertension
- Diabetes
- Tobacco smoking or hyperlipidemia
- Vasculitis or hypercoagulable states (young patients, age <40–50)

## Stroke: Fast Hit Summary

- What is stroke?
  - Sudden neurological deficit
- How does it present?
  - Most often unilateral weakness of both upper and lower extremity
  - Speech and visual defects common
- What testing is needed?
  - Echo, carotid Doppler, EKG, and telemetry in almost all patients
- What is treatment?
  - **No** treatment until stat head CT excludes blood!
  - Thrombolytics in first 3–4.5 hours after onset in some
  - After 3–4.5 hours use aspirin, clopidogrel, or aspirin with dipyridamole
  - Rehabilitation evaluation for physical & occupational therapy

## Presentation

### Middle Cerebral Artery (MCA)

- Weakness on one side of the body (opposite side of stroke)
- Sparing of the upper part of the face (forehead)
- Pronator drift on one side (subtle motor weakness)

- Visual field loss on side of weakness (homonymous hemianopsia)
- Sensory loss

### Anterior Cerebral Artery

- Psychiatric/personal changes
- Weakness: legs > arms
- Urinary incontinence
- Testing and treatment identical to MCA stroke

### Posterior (Vertebrobasilar) Circulation Stroke Syndromes

- Loss of consciousness *only* from posterior circulation
- Altered mental status/dizziness
- Bilateral deficits *only* from posterior circulation, e.g., cranial nerve or sensory disturbance on one side and weakness or ataxia on the other

**Posterior circulation = brainstem and/or cerebellum**

Posterior circulation will cause:

- Dysarthria
- Dysphagia
- Dizziness
- Diplopia

## Diagnostic Testing

To see if stroke has occurred, do the following

1. Head CT without contrast: blood shows **instantly**; embolic at 3–4 days
2. MRA: positive as early as 1–2 hours
3. MRI: embolic (nonbloody) at 24 hours

MRI/MRA is indispensible for posterior stroke.

To find the reason for stroke, do the following:

- Echocardiogram
- EKG/telemetry
- Carotid duplex U/S for MCA and anterior stroke
  - Carotid study *is not useful* for posterior stroke

**Round Saver**

Look at the head CT yourself.

When evaluating for vasculitis/thrombophilia, look for young patients (age <40–50) with no risks (hypertension, diabetes, tobacco, lipid):

- ANA, ESR, VDRL or RPR, CRP
- Factor V Leiden, protein C/S, antiphospholipid antibody, antithrombin

## Treatment

- If <3–4.5 hours: thrombolytics (tPA)
  - If too late for tPA: aspirin
- If already on aspirin with the stroke: switch to clopidogrel or add dipyridamole
- To prevent recurrence:
  - If carotid >70–99% stenosis: surgical endarterectomy
  - If atrial fibrillation/flutter: warfarin, dabigatran, or rivaroxaban
  - If echo shows clot: warfarin

**How NOT to Kill Your Patient**

Several treatments are dangerous in CVA—all increase the risk of bleeding:

- Heparin
- tPA when >4.5 hours post-stroke
- Combined aspirin **and** clopidogrel
- Prasugrel

# Delirium/Confusion

Delirium is an "altered level of sensorium." It is not just a memory problem like dementia. Synonyms for delirium are lethargy, obtundation, altered mental status, and stupor.

> **Round Saver**
>
> Delirium is like being drunk.

Problems/abnormalities that lead to delirium can also cause seizures when they are severe enough.

## Diagnostic Testing

The following lab tests MUST be checked before going on rounds with your attending. Do not allow yourself to be caught saying, "Oops, I did not check."

- Hypoxia
- Hypoglycemia
- Sodium: both high and low
- Calcium: high creates lethargy, low creates seizures
- Liver or renal failure
- Magnesium (rare)

If the above tests are normal, proceed to check the following:

- Urine toxicology: opiates, benzodiazepines, barbiturates, cocaine
- Head CT/MRI
- CNS infection of any kind (meningitis, encephalitis)

Remember that seizures can also cause confusion. If all of the tests above are normal and no cause of seizure is found, get an EEG.

# Seizures

Do not restrain or hold down anyone having a seizure. It does not stop the seizing and only leads to dislocation of joints.

**Round Saver**

If your patient is seizing, get help immediately.

With acute seizure:

1. **Get help.** If you are first to arrive, get the nurse/support staff to call your resident. Call a "Seizure Code" or alert the "Rapid Response Team" if your hospital has one. This is because *you cannot write medication orders* that the patient will need.
2. **Pad the area** around the patient to avoid self-injury if they "flail around."
3. **Send labs** (oxygen, glucose, sodium, calcium, magnesium, LFTs, creatinine, urine toxicology screen).
4. **Start oxygen and IV fluids** if not already done.
5. **Start drug therapy**, benzodiazepine IV to start.

**Round Saver**

Noncompliance with AED very commonly causes seizures.

## Status Epilepticus: Emergency Drug Therapy

**"Status epilepticus" = persistent seizure not resolving spontaneously**

1. Benzodiazepine:
    - Lorazepam (Ativan) 2 mg IV push
    - Repeat Ativan 2 mg IV push in 5 minutes or less if still seizing
    - Give Ativan 2–3 times then go onto fosphenytoin
2. Fosphenytoin IV
3. Phenobarbital

4. General anesthesia: Get patient to ICU!
    - Prepare to intubate!
    - Midazolam
    - Propofol
    - Pentobarbital or thiopental

## Long-Term Antiepileptic Drug (AED) Use

### Who Does Not Need AEDs?

- Do not treat most **first-time, single seizures**.
- Do not use long-term AEDs for **alcohol-related seizures**.
- Do not use AED for seizures from the metabolic or toxin-related disorders described above. In these cases, fix the disorder (e.g., calcium, glucose, oxygen).

### Who Should Be Treated?

- Those presenting in **status epilepticus**
- **Abnormal EEG**
- Uncorrectable cause (e.g., brain tumor)
- Strong **family history**

### Choice of AED

There is no clear first choice for AED long term. Phenytoin, valproic acid, levetiracetam (Keppra), carbamazepine, Lamotrigine, and several others can all be used first.

**Round Saver**

AED choice depends on attending's preference.

1. If AED noncompliance or low blood level caused the seizure, just restart the medication and discharge patient home
2. If compliant with AED and blood level is in therapeutic range, ask attending, "Do you want to add a second AED or switch?"
3. No clear best first choice in pregnancy

4. No clear duration of AED or when you can stop. Must go for at least 1–2 years without seizures

Rules on driving vary state to state. Regardless of AED chosen, tell the patient not to drive.

## HEADACHE

Your first job is to make sure the patient's headache is not from serious pathology such as:

- Hemorrhagic stroke/subarachnoid hemorrhage (SAH)
- Tumor/mass

Order CT first. MRI is the best test.

### Who to Scan?

- New-onset severe headache
- Focal neurological deficits
- Seizure
- Papilledema
- Confusion/altered mental status

If the patient has long-term, repetitive headaches with a diagnosis of migraine or cluster headache, you do not need to scan the patient.

# Migraine Headache

There is no diagnostic test for migraine. It is based on a symptom complex characterized by visual disturbance. Migraine patients often "feel it coming on" or see an "aura."

- Flashing lights
- Floating "black dots" or "scotoma"
- Photophobia

- Can be either unilateral or bilateral
- Very rarely leads to focal neurological deficit

The association with foods (chocolate, red wine, cheese) and menstruation is real. This is not just something they made you memorize for your Step 1 exam.

## Cluster Headache

- Symptom complex: multiple, brief, intense episodes over short period of time
- Occurrence: men > women
- Eye: red, tearing, rhinorrhea

**Round Saver**

Migraine: bad visual problem

Cluster: eye looks bad

### Treatment of Migraine and Cluster Headache

1. Triptans (e.g., sumatriptan) or ergotamine to abort acute headache
   - Cluster also aborted with 100% oxygen
2. Prophylaxis:
   - Migraine: propranolol
   - Cluster: verapamil

Triptans are contraindicated in those with coronary disease or severe uncontrolled hypertension, and in pregnant women. There are numerous alternatives to propranolol for prophylaxis such as phenytoin, carbamazepine, valproic acid, SSRIs, or pregabalin. None of them is clearly superior.

## CENTRAL NERVOUS SYSTEM (CNS) INFECTIONS

CNS infections have:

- Fever
- Headache
- Sometimes nausea, vomiting, seizure

It is often not clear until after the lumbar puncture whether meningitis is present.

### What to Ask About

- "Do the lights bother your eyes?"
- "Do you feel confused? Is it hard for you to think straight?"
- "Does your neck feel stiff?"

### Who Needs Antibiotics before LP?

When patients come with CNS infections, some will need a CT scan of the head before an LP can be safely done. In these cases, antibiotics should be given first. Immediately administer ceftriaxone, vancomycin, and dexamethasone if there are signs of meningitis (fever, headache, stiff neck) and:

- Focal neurological findings
- Seizures
- Severe confusion (makes neurological examination inaccurate)
- Papilledema

## Meningitis

1. Look for neck stiffness and photophobia
2. Determine if CT is needed before LP (focal/seizure/severe confusion)
3. If CT needed, give antibiotics
   - Ceftriaxone 2 g + vancomycin 1 g every 12 hours plus dexamethasone
   - Add ampicillin 2 g every 4 hours if elderly or immunocompromised
4. If CT not needed, get LP done within 30–60 minutes
5. Use CSF cell count to identify meningitis
   - Thousands of PMNs = bacterial
6. Get CSF protein level, Gram stain, and cultures—but these are less helpful in the urgent treatment decision than cell count and differential
   - Protein level can be high in almost every form of meningitis
   - Normal CSF protein excludes bacterial meningitis
   - Gram useful if positive, worthless if negative
   - Culture takes 2–3 days—too long in acute treatment decision
7. Antigen detection:
   - Like a Gram stain: latex testing for specific antigen
   - Specific if positive, useless if negative
   - Used in those getting antibiotics prior to LP

**How NOT to Kill Your Patient**

In CNS infections, antibiotics continue until bacterial infection is excluded.

| CSF Analysis | | | |
|---|---|---|---|
| **Feature in History/ Physical** | **Organism** | **Test** | **Treatment** |
| Lung lesions, immigrant | Tuberculosis | High protein, culture<br>3 high-volume CSF samples—centrifuge them! | Rifampin, isoniazid, pyrazinamide, ethambutol steroids |
| AIDS, CD4 <100 | Cryptococcus | Antigen >95% sensitive | Amphotericin + 5FC |
| Camper/hiker, rash, joint | Lyme | Western blot, PCR, serology | Ceftriaxone |
| Tick (60%) rash wrist/ankles moves to body | Rickettsia | Western blot, PCR, serology | Doxycycline |
| None | Viral | None | None |

## Encephalitis

**Acute fever + confusion = encephalitis**

- Neck stiffness and photophobia sometimes accompany encephalitis
- Skin or genital lesions do not always accompany herpes encephalitis
- PCR for herpes simplex is the most accurate test (even better than brain biopsy)
- CT before LP because of confusion
- Look for few hundred lymphocytes on CSF
- Add acyclovir (10 mg/kg) to ceftriaxone/vancomycin until CT and LP determine etiology
- Do not worry about short-term (3–5 days) use of steroids if the diagnosis is unclear

## Brain Abscess

You cannot tell the content of a mass lesion in the brain from CT or MRI alone, because cancer and infection both show "ring" or "contrast enhancement" on CT/MRI. Next steps:

- HIV-negative patients need a brain biopsy.
- HIV-positive patients can be treated for toxoplasmosis and have the scan repeated.

> **Round Saver**
>
> Do not shift care of the patient around logistics.

Transfer the patient if needed in order to get the biopsy. Pissing off staff/attending to get the care the patient needs is a virtue!

**Do not** let anyone plan for 6 weeks of empiric therapy for brain abscess:

1. You cannot be sure whether the ring-enhancing lesion is an infection or a cancer.
2. Infection (abscess) has such a broad range of organisms, you will never be sure you are covering the right organism!

## Subarachnoid Hemorrhage (SAH)

- Fever/headache/stiff neck/photophobia
- Onset more sudden than in meningitis, but can be VERY similar
- Loss of consciousness (LOC) in 50% from increased intracranial pressure
- Focal neurological abnormalities 30%

**Sudden onset meningitis + LOC = subarachnoid**

## Diagnostic Testing

1. Head CT: 95% sensitive on first day; CT loses 5% sensitivity per day
2. If CT is negative, do an LP
3. Blood on CSF or xanthochromia is diagnostic
4. Angiography determines the location so you can repair it. It does not diagnose the SAH.

## Treatment

1. Embolize the site of bleeding with platinum wire delivered by catheter placed into the cerebral vasculature. This is superior to a surgically placed clip, which requires brain surgery.
2. Give nimodipine, a calcium channel blocker to prevent recurrences. After the aneurysm ruptures and the vessel bleeds there is vasospasm that can lead to a stroke. Nimodipine prevents this stroke.
3. If hydrocephalus develops, a ventriculoperitoneal shunt needs to be placed.

# Guillain-Barré Syndrome (GBS)

- Weakness in the lower extremities starting in feet moving up toward chest
- Loss/absence of deep tendon reflexes (DTRs) of legs
- Can follow gastroenteritis with organisms like *Campylobacter* or rarely EBV
- Death from respiratory failure occurs when weakness hits diaphragm
- Assess respiratory function with PFTs (FVC)
- Look for decreased peak *inspiratory* pressure

**Ascending weakness + loss of reflexes = GBS**

## Diagnostic Testing

1. Pulmonary function testing to assess possibility of respiratory involvement
2. Nerve conduction velocity decrease is most accurate
3. High CSF protein with no WBCs of limited use

## Treatment

1. Intravenous immunoglobulin (IVIG)
2. Plasmapheresis

> **Round Saver**
>
> IVIG is easier to use than plasmapheresis and just as effective in GBS. Steroids don't help!!

# Dementia

Dementia from Alzheimer's disease (AD) is often present in patients admitted to a medical service. It is hard for staff to pay attention to this component of the patient's illness when they are focusing on the MI, PE, or CHF exacerbation that is acutely life threatening. You, as the student, may be the only person to bring attention to this area.

> **Round Saver**
>
> Vivid visual hallucinations are found most in Lewy body dementia. Frontotemporal loses social skills first!

## Alzheimer's Disease (AD)

AD is a progressive memory disorder found almost exclusively in those above age 65.

- Focal neurological abnormalities are rare
- Head CT/MRI shows atrophy
- B12, VDRL/RPR, and thyroid function should be confirmed as normal
- LP is not necessary

## Treatment

1. Acetylcholinesterase inhibitors are first-line therapy (they are equal):
   - Rivastigmine
   - Galantamine
   - Donepezil
2. Neuroprotective medication:
   - Memantine

**Dementia Syndromes Other Than Alzheimer's Disease**

| Dementia Syndrome | Unique Feature | Test/Treatment |
|---|---|---|
| Lewy body | Parkinson's disease (PD)<br>Hallucinations, fluctuations in cognition | No specific test<br>Treat with AD and PD drugs |
| Frontotemporal | Social appropriateness lost first<br>Earlier than AD (50–60)<br>Hygiene issues, disinhibition, lack of tact or etiquette | Lobar atrophy on scan<br>AD drugs<br>Antipsychotic meds |
| Creutzfeldt-Jakob | Rapid progression over months<br>Myoclonus | 14-3-3 protein on CSF<br>No treatment |
| Normal pressure hydrocephalus | Urinary incontinence, ataxia | Head scan, shunt |
| Huntington's disease | Emotional lability<br>Movement disorder (chorea) | CAG trinucleotide repeats<br>Tetrabenazine treatment |
| Multi-infarct | Sudden deteriorations in stepwise fashion | MRI, treat stroke |

AD drugs = acetylcholinesterase inhibitors and memantine

# Multiple Sclerosis (MS)

- Admitted for sudden decompensation with increased weakness needing high-dose steroids
- No test assesses/confirms exacerbation; all clinically based: "Do you feel weaker?"
- Optic neuritis = sudden unilateral vision decrease/loss confirmed by eye exam

## Presentation

MS presents a defect at any level of the CNS. The most common manifestation is optic neuritis, but it can be motor (weakness) or sensory. Fatigue—just feeling "out of gas"—is very common, as are painful muscles from spasticity. MS is extremely uncomfortable and very depressing for patients. There is no cure.

> **Round Saver**
>
> In internuclear ophthalmoplegia, one eye gets stuck at midline, one eye has nystagmus.

## Diagnostic Testing

1. MRI: first and most accurate test
2. CSF: "oligoclonal bands" only occasionally needed if MRI is equivocal (rare, <3%)

## Treatment

1. High-dose glucocorticoids (methylprednisolone IV 1,000 mg daily for 3 days)
2. Delay progression with
   - Beta interferon
   - Glatiramer
   - Mitoxantrone

- Natalizumab (causes progressive multifocal leukoencephalopathy)
- Fingolimod (only oral drug for MS)
- Dalfampridine (increases walking speed)

### Disease Manifestations and Treatment

| Manifestation | Treatment |
| --- | --- |
| Fatigue | Amantadine |
| Neurogenic bladder (atonic) | Urecholine (bethanechol) |
| Spasticity | Baclofen, tizanidine |
| Urge incontinence | Oxybutynin, tolterodine |

## Head Trauma

Head trauma is common but rarely leads to focal arm or leg weakness. Concussion alone cannot cause focal neurological defects. Order CT to evaluate head trauma that is severe enough to result in confusion or loss of consciousness (LOC).

**LOC = CT**

You cannot tell whether someone has an epidural hematoma, subdural hematoma, or contusion from history and physical examination alone.

- All head trauma can cause LOC or altered mental status
- Focal neurological abnormalities exclude a simple concussion
- "Lucid interval" = LOC, then awakening, followed several hours later by second LOC
- It is impossible to distinguish epidural from subdural hematoma without a CT scan

**Round Saver**

"Lucid interval" is found in both subdural and epidural.

- CT is better than MRI for blood
- Head trauma causes EKG abnormalities ("cerebral T-waves")

There is no treatment for concussion. Most patients diagnosed with concussion can go home from the emergency department.

### Intracranial Bleeding Management

- Small, minor bleeds with no signs of compression should not be drained
- PPIs are stress ulcer prophylaxis in all head trauma
- Large bleeds with midline shift need:
  - Intubation for hyperventilation to rapidly decrease intracranial pressure
  - Place in ICU
  - Emergency neurosurgery and neurology evaluation
  - Possible evacuation

> **Round Saver**
> Large brain bleed from trauma should be on surgery service!

## Back Pain and Cord Compression

The vast majority of back pain is minor and needs no treatment beyond analgesics such as NSAIDs and modest stretching/exercise. Do not do routine spine imaging such as an MRI.

> **Round Saver**
> Abnormal "straight leg raise" is **not** compression!

Cord compression, on the other hand, is a neurosurgical/neurological emergency and needs instant administration of steroids to prevent permanent paralysis. High-dose dexamethasone is given **stat** for:

- Hyperreflexia
- Upgoing toes (extensor plantar reflex)

- Bilateral lower extremity weakness
- Sensory "level": decreased pain perception below a certain nerve root level
- Vertebral tenderness
- Urine and bowel incontinence

### Summary of Back Pain

Low back muscle strain:

- Pain and "soreness" is common and needs no imaging.
- No MRI, no bed rest.

Cord compression:

- Emergency neurological disaster needing immediate high-dose steroids (dexamethasone)/MRI
- Increased DTRs, upgoing toes, sensory level, weakness, vertebral tenderness

> **Round Saver**
>
> Delay on compression = paralysis.

## Parkinson's Disease (PD)

Parkinson's disease is a gait disorder with orthostasis and tremor.

Those with PD usually have a visible tremor and all their movements are slow with rigidity. There are no specific tests, so the diagnosis and the intensity of treatment are entirely based on the severity of the disability.

### Things You Will Be Asked on Rounds

- Problem walking. Is it difficult to walk across the street before the light changes?
  - PD is a severe gait disorder
- Lightheadedness rising from a chair or bed
  - Orthostasis is common
- Shaking of the hands. Does shaking get better or worse when reaching for things?
  - PD is a resting tremor
- Change in size of writing
  - Micrographia
- Medications for a psychiatric issue
  - PD is an adverse effect of many antipsychotic medications as an "extrapyramidal symptom"
- Medications for dementia or memory; recent dose increase
  - Dementia medication worsens or provokes PD
- Recent comments by family/friends about seeming unemotional or cold
  - Hypomimia

## Treatment

With **mild disease**, tremor is the main issue. Treat with:

- **Anticholinergic medication**
  - Benztropine, trihexyphenidyl
  - Contraindicated with older patients because of adverse effects
    - Constipation
    - Urine retention
    - Glaucoma
    - Worsening dementia

- **Amantadine**
  - Mildly effective, but few adverse effects

With **severe disease**, gait disorder and orthostasis become more severe. Use:

- Direct-acting dopamine agonists
  - Ropinirole, pramipexole
  - Less efficacy and fewer adverse effects
- Levodopa/carbidopa
  - More efficacy
  - "On/off" phenomena: dopamine need varies and meds can be too much (dyskinesia) or too little (locked in immobility)
- COMT inhibitor
  - Tolcapone, entacapone
  - Only as "add-on" to levodopa/carbidopa
- MAO inhibitor
  - Selegiline, rasagiline
  - Not clear precisely when to use

Note that PD medications cause psychosis, and psychosis medications cause PD. Similarly, dementia medications worsen PD, and PD medications worsen dementia.

1. Antipsychotic medications inhibit dopamine. Inhibiting dopamine leads to PD symptoms or worsens them in those with the diagnosis.
2. Dementia medications such as donepezil, rivastigmine, and galantamine increase acetylcholine to increase memory. PD is treated with anticholinergic medications (benztropine, trihexyphenidyl). Dementia medications worsen PD.
3. PD medications inhibit acetylcholine, so they worsen dementia.
4. PD medications increase dopamine (ropinirole, pramipexole) or replace dopamine (levodopa/carbidopa). Increased dopamine causes psychosis in as much as 40% of those with PD.

## Restless Legs Syndrome

- Uncomfortable feeling in legs at night
- "Creepy-crawly feeling" relieved by moving the legs
- Frequently kicks bed partner
- Associated with iron deficiency for unclear reasons
- Treat with ropinirole, pramipexole

## Essential Tremor

- Isolated tremor with no associated physical or laboratory abnormalities
- Tremor at both rest and with exertion
- Treat with propranolol
- Other therapies are: primidone, alcohol, and benzodiazepines

## Amyotrophic Lateral Sclerosis (ALS)

- Idiopathic destruction of motor neurons
- Affects both upper and lower motor neurons
- No specific test
- Riluzole is only drug to decrease progression

| Upper Motor Defects | Lower Motor Defects |
|---|---|
| Spasticity<br>Hyperreflexia<br>Upgoing toes (extensor plantar reflexes) | Wasting<br>Fasciculations<br>Gait disorder |

### Management of Respiratory Issues in ALS

- Daytime somnolence managed at first with CPAP and BiPAP
- Tracheostomy needed later
- Severe disease needs ventilator use at night

## Peripheral Neuropathy/ Postherpetic Neuralgia

This is a very frustrating disorder. Patients are very uncomfortable, and no therapy is fully effective.

- "Burning, numbness, tingling"
- Most common cause: diabetes, herpes zoster
- Most accurate test: nerve conduction studies
- Best initial therapy: pregabalin, gabapentin, venlafaxane, amitriptyline

## Trigeminal Neuralgia

- Idiopathic pain disorder of CN5
- Exclusively sensory disturbance
- Severe, "like being stabbed in the face with a knife"
- Brought on by chewing, touching the face
- Best initial therapy: carbamazepine
- Alternates: oxcarbazepine, valproic acid
- Surgical "rhizotomy" if medical therapy fails: cut the nerve or inject alcohol to "ablate" the nerve

## Myasthenia Gravis

This disorder is rarely admitted to the hospital. Look for people who feel weak—this is not the same thing as fatigue. Myasthenia is a direct muscular weakness, and it noticeably worsens at the end of the day.

### Presentation

- Double vision (extraocular muscles get weak)
- Decreased ability to chew, worse toward the end of meals
- Weakness with repetitive use of muscles

### Diagnostic Testing

1. First: acetylcholine receptor antibodies
2. Most accurate: single fiber electromyography (EMG)
3. Chest imaging to exclude thymoma and thymic hyperplasia
4. Neurology consultation (on boards, however, never consult on rare disorders like myasthenia)

**Round Saver**

Edrophonium (Tensilon) testing is the most common wrong answer! Its use is largely historical.

### Treatment

Patients in acute myasthenic crisis can be admitted with a sudden, overwhelming generalized muscular weakness. Respiratory involvement and placement in the ICU or on a ventilator are particularly dangerous.

- Intravenous immunoglobulin or plasmapheresis
- Glucocorticoids in high doses intravenously

### Chronic Disease Management

1. Acetylcholinesterase inhibitor: pyridostigmine or neostigmine
2. If it progresses:
   - Thymectomy in those <60–70 years old
   - Prednisone in older persons (>60–70)
3. Steroid-sparing medications: used long term to get patients off steroids so that the immune defect is suppressed
   - Cyclosporine
   - Cyclophosphamide
   - Tacrolimus, sirolimus
   - Mycophenolate
   - Azathioprine/6MP

## Spinal Cord Disorders

| Disorder | Characteristic Feature |
|---|---|
| Subacute combined degeneration | Loss of position and vibratory sense<br>$B_{12}$ deficiency, syphilis |
| Anterior spinal artery infarction | Retaining only position/vibratory sense<br>Everything else (sensory, motor, touch) lost |
| Syringomyelia | Pain & temperature lost bilaterally<br>Across both arms “capelike” distribution<br>MRI and surgical repair |
| Brown-Séquard (hemisection of cord) | Pain & temperature loss: contralateral<br>Position & vibratory loss: unilateral |

# Preventive Medicine 8

## CANCER SCREENING

Only 3 screening methods are clearly beneficial in the prevention of cancer: breast, cervical, and colon.

### Breast Cancer

Breast cancer is extremely common in women, affecting about 1 in 9. Mammography is used to screen. There has been considerable controversy over the recommended time for the *first* mammography. The greatest benefit is at age >50, but a number of professional organizations recommend starting at age 40. Attending physicians often disagree on the age to start mammography, so ask your attending his or her personal preference.

> **Round Saver**
>
> Mammography: Ask your attending her preferences.

What is clear, however, is that if you screen the general population, you detect many more treatable cancers and have a much greater mortality benefit above age 50. Mammography must begin by age 50.

Prophylaxis can prevent high-risk patients from getting breast cancer in the first place. Tamoxifen can decrease breast cancer by 30–50% in high-risk patients, i.e., those with 2 first-degree relatives who have had breast cancer. In these patients, tamoxifen should be started at age 35–40. The benefit is not as clear with raloxifene.

BRCA confuses students. We don't know what to do if it is positive. Prophylactic mastectomy is a lot harder to handle than prophylactic tamoxifen.

**Round Saver**

Don't be surprised if your resident has not heard that tamoxifen prevents breast cancer!

Protecting patients is more important than protecting your grade.

## Cervical Cancer

- Start screening at age 21
- Age of onset of sexual activity has no bearing on these recommendations
- Pap every 3 years for ages 21–65
- For ages 30–65, either
  - Pap smear every 3 years **OR**
  - Pap **and HPV testing** combined **every 5 years**

## Colon Cancer

95% of colon cancer is preventable with proper screening.

- General population:
  - Start at age 50
  - Colonoscopy every 10 years
- One first-degree relative (parent or sibling)
  - Start at age 40 or 10 years earlier than when family member had colon cancer, whichever is earlier
  - Colonoscopy every 10 years if family member was age >60
  - Colonoscopy every 5 years if family member was age <60
- Polyp found on colonoscopy
  - Repeat colonoscopy in 3–5 years

### Other Cancer Screening

There are several other screening methods for cancer that might do something but are not clearly effective. Preventive medicine recommendations can change rapidly if guidelines are published. At present, therefore, the following tests ***cannot*** be recommended as standard screening methods:

- Chest x-ray
- BRCA
- Prostate-specific antigen (PSA): not recommended
- Pelvic ultrasound: there is no clearly beneficial screen for ovarian cancer
- Chest CT: benefit is unclear, even in smokers

## Abdominal Aortic Aneurysm (AAA)

- Screen men if current or former tobacco smokers
- Age >65
- Once with an ultrasound

There is no routine screening for carotid stenosis.

## Osteoporosis

- Screen all women age >65
- DEXA bone densitometry

**Round Saver**

Remember, you went to medical school to help people.

## Hypertension, Lipid Disturbances, and Diabetes

Recommendations on screening for hypertension, lipid disturbances, and diabetes are very unclear. That is because, on a Medicine Ward or clerkship rotation, you will only see patients already being tested for these issues. Thus, you cannot do a study withholding what is routine care for every patient.

In a health care facility, everyone you see will have had their blood pressure checked. For inpatients, glucose testing is universal.

The clearest evidence for screening is:

- Blood pressure every visit for every patient age >18
- LDL measurement:
  - Men age >35 every 5 years
  - Women age >45 every 5 years
  - Earlier if there are risk factors such as diabetes or hypertension
- Diabetes (2 fasting glucoses or HbA1c):
  - Anyone hypertensive or obese

## Smoking

- Ask all patients if they smoke
- Advise them to stop
- Assist with setting a quit date
- Arrange follow-up to make sure they quit.
- Assist with medications, education is not sufficient.
  - Bupropion and varenicline are the most effective.
  - Nicotine patch is more effective than nicotine gum.

**Round Saver** 

Save a life! Help someone stop smoking.

## Alcoholism

Alcoholism must be treated as a disease even if you or your supervising physician sees it as a moral or "willpower" failure. The only model that produces results addresses the chemical dependency as an obsession of the mind and a physical dependence.

The **CAGE** questions are accurate and effective. Ask the patient:

- Cut down: "Are you trying or do you want to cut down the amount of alcohol you drink?"
- Angry/annoyed: "Do you feel angry or annoyed because I am asking about your drinking?"
- Guilty: "Do you feel guilty about how much you drink?"
- Eye opener: "Do you need to have a drink to 'get started' in the morning?"

Remember, alcoholism is a self-diagnosed disease. People do not "feel good" about themselves because they are alcoholic; there is a deep sense of shame and self-loathing. You are helping people become happy by asking them these questions, even if they feel annoyed at the moment when you are asking. Ask the patient if he or she wants help getting sober.

## Domestic Violence and Suicide Prevention

- Ask every patient about these things; don't expect people to volunteer this information
- You do not have the right to report the information without patient consent
- 750 people a week successfully commit suicide in the United States! Find them before it is too late.

Preventive medicine guidelines can change instantly.

# Vaccinations

## Adult Immunization

| Vaccine | Indication |
|---|---|
| *Streptococcus pneumoniae* | • Age >65<br>• Chronic illness<br>◦ COPD, asthma<br>◦ HIV positive, steroid use, diabetes mellitus<br>◦ Lymphoma or any leukemia<br>◦ Asplenia or primary immunodeficiency<br>◦ Chronic liver or kidney disease<br>◦ Cochlear implants |
| Varicella zoster (shingles) | Age >60, 1x |
| Influenza | Any age, 1x/year |
| Tetanus | • Every 10 years routinely<br>• In 5 years if wound is "dirty" |
| Hepatitis B | • Healthcare profession<br>• Blood product recipient<br>• Chronic liver disease<br>• Sexually promiscuity |
| Hepatitis A | • Travel to places where water/food is not safe<br>• Chronic liver disease |

The varicella vaccine is not safe in pregnancy. The hepatitis vaccines are most helpful in those with baseline liver disease.

Everyone should get a Tdap (tetanus, diphtheria, acellular pertussis) as at least one of the tetanus boosters.

## Post-Exposure Prophylaxis (PEP)

| Exposure | Prophylaxis |
|---|---|
| HIV needle-stick | 2 nucleosides and 1 protease inhibitor for 1 month |
| Hepatitis B | If no protective antibody: hepatitis B immunoglobulin and vaccine |
| Varicella | If no protective antibody: varicella immunoglobulin and vaccine |
| Rabies | Rabies immune globulin and vaccine |

Note that a bat bite is not required for transmission of rabies. Just being in the same room as a bat is sufficient!

# Pulmonology 9

## Shortness of Breath or Dyspnea

Since a number of conditions can make it hard to get enough air, you must collect an accurate patient history to narrow down possible causes of dyspnea.

### Things You Will Be Asked on Rounds

- Speed of onset
- Chest pain
- If pain changes with respiration (pleuritic)
- If shortness of breath gets better or worse with walking
- If breathing improves with sitting up
- History of asthma or emphysema (COPD)
- Previous clots in the legs
- Previously struck in the chest
- Sleepiness during the day

## Etiology

| History | Associated with |
|---|---|
| Sudden onset | PE, pneumothorax, asthma exacerbation |
| Pleuritic | Pneumonia, PE, pneumothorax, pleuritis |
| Improves with sitting up | CHF |
| Clots in legs | Pulmonary embolus (PE) |
| Nonpleuritic pain | Coronary disease/myocardial infarction |
| Trauma, asthma/COPD | Pneumothorax, tamponade |
| Daytime somnolence | Sleep apnea |

"Pleuritic" pain changes with respiration; PE = pulmonary embolus

## Diagnostic Testing

Expect to get or see these tests on all patients with dyspnea:

- Oximetry
- Arterial blood gas (when severe, acute, and in hospital)
- Chest x-ray

The oximeter is extremely accurate at determining the oxygen saturation. Oximetry on a finger or toe will be within 1–2% of the level measured on an arterial blood gas (ABG). Severe hypoxia is <90% saturation.

Although oxygen saturation of >95% excludes severe lung disease, the oximeter cannot tell you:

- pH
- $pCO_2$
- Alveolar-arterial (A-a) gradient

For instance, the oximeter cannot reliably distinguish $pO_2$ of 65 mmHg from $pO_2$ of 85 mmHg. This is because oxygen saturation rises >90% at $pO_2$ of 60 mmHg and will be 95% saturated by $pO_2$ of 70 mmHg. Thus, the oximeter cannot reveal *how hard the patient is working* to achieve that saturation.

The normal respiratory rate is 10–14 breaths/minute. If a person breathes very fast to keep his oxygen saturation >90%, he will tire out and be in danger.

Consider the following 2 patients with $pO_2$ of 70 mmHg, saturation 95%:

**Round Saver**

You will always be asked on rotation *why* your patient is on oxygen. Don't give oxygen without knowing why it is needed.

| | Patient 1 | Patient 2 |
|---|---|---|
| $pO_2$ | 70 | 70 |
| Sat | 95% | 95% |
| RR | 12 | 24 |
| $pCO_2$ | 40 | 20 |
| pH | 7.4 | 7.56 |
| A-a | 30 | 55 |

With a fast respiration rate and very high A-a gradient, Patient 2 is much sicker than Patient 1. As this example demonstrates, very severe hypoxia can be present with an oxygen saturation that *looks* safely above 90–95%. Dyspneic patients with saturation of 90–95% need an ABG.

Technical considerations for ABG:

- Transport the ABG on ice
- Get it to the lab fast

## Guidelines for Oximeter and ABG Interpretation

To interpret the oximetry or ABG results, you must know *how much oxygen was used to get there.* It is not sufficient to say "The saturation is normal." In an older patient with COPD, a $pO_2$ of

70 mmHg and saturation of 95% on room air is excellent. The same values on 50% face mask mean the patient is very ill. In the second scenario, it is like saying "I have $50,000 in my pocket" but neglecting to add "because I sold my house and maximized my credit cards."

**Round Saver** 

Know the ABG results on dyspneic patients.

Oximetry and ABG readings are easiest to interpret when done on room air. Recording that the $pO_2$ is 70 is not as meaningful as saying "The $pO_2$ is 70 while breathing room air."

**How NOT to Kill Your Patient**

- Oximetry is first in all patients with dyspnea
- Saturation >90% is acceptable for life
- Saturation >90% does not exclude serious lung disease
- You must know how much oxygen is being used to interpret results
- ABG is far more accurate than oximetry
- Alveolar-arterial gradient is essential in all severely ill dyspneic patients

Know the amount of oxygen being used in all dyspneic patients. Shortness of breath is so intrinsic and common to the Internal Medicine service that if you do not master the ABG, you cannot truly "master the Wards."

**Round Saver** 

Dyspnea automatically means instability. Know *why* the patient is dyspneic.

### Alveolar-arterial (A-a) Gradient

On room air, alveolar oxygen = 150 mmHg:

$$150 - (pCO_2/0.8 + pO_2)$$

A-a gradients gradually increase as we age. An A-a gradient of 15–20 would be normal in a person age >70–80. The average increase in A-a gradient is about 1 point for every 5 years of age.

As a student, you will assume the patient is on oxygen for a reason determined by all the senior people above you. I strongly encourage you **not** to trust anyone. Confirm for yourself the reason for oxygen use. The attending may just not be paying attention.

## PNEUMONIA

Pneumonia is the most common infectious cause of death in the United States, yet 80% of patients can be treated in the outpatient setting. All forms of pneumonia present with fever and cough. Severe infection is associated with dyspnea.

> **Round Saver**
>
> Make sure you look at the x-ray yourself, even if you can't understand it.

### Things You Will Be Asked on Rounds

- Diagnosis: fever, cough, sputum, chest x-ray
- Severity: Has BP, pulse oximeter, or ABG been checked?
- Placement: CURB65
  - Confusion
  - Uremia
  - Respiratory distress
  - BP low
  - Age >65
- Treatment: Was first dose of antibiotics given?

The following diseases predispose patients to more pneumonia and worsening severity of illness.

- Chronic obstructive pulmonary disease (COPD)
- Liver or renal disease
- Cancer, diabetes, or chronic heart disease
- Alcoholism, asplenia, or immunosuppression

## Community-Acquired Pneumonia (CAP)

No matter what city your rotation is in, you will see CAP. CAP is a disease *you must know*. The most common cause is still pneumococcus.

The majority of patients with CAP will not have an identifiable cause: CAP simply "happens." Look for a patient with cough, fever, and shortness of breath. Some patients will have sputum production. Discolored sputum in indicative of bacterial infection, but you can't say which one—you cannot correlate colors of sputum with a specific organism.

### Things You Will Be Asked on Rounds

| Point of history | Disease to suspect |
|---|---|
| AIDS with CD4 <200 | Pneumocystis |
| Recent immigration | Tuberculosis |
| Diarrhea, abdominal pain | Legionella |
| Bird exposure | *Chlamydia psittaci* |
| River valleys | Histoplasmosis |
| Dry cough | Mycoplasma, chlamydia, coxiella, legionella, viruses |

## Diagnostic Testing

- Oximeter and ABG to assess severity of CAP
- Chest x-ray
- Sputum stain and culture if sputum is produced
- BUN and creatinine to assess severity

To determine where to place the patient, use the following guidelines.

- **Mild:**
    - No hypoxia or confusion, normal BP
    - **Discharge home on oral antibiotics**
- **Moderate:**
    - Mild hypoxia, borderline low systolic blood pressure (SBP) (90–110 mmHg), age >65
    - **Regular hospital ward**
- **Severe:**
    - SBP <90 mmHg after fluids
    - Tachycardia
    - $pO_2$ <60 despite 2–4 liters nasal cannula
    - **Intensive care unit**

## Treatment of CAP

| Comorbidity or Recent Antibiotic Use | Outpatient | Regular Hospital Ward | Intensive Care Unit |
|---|---|---|---|
| No | Azithromycin or clarithromycin | • Ceftriaxone or cefotaxime<br>**and**<br>• Azithromycin or clarithromycin | Ceftriaxone, cefotaxime, ertapenem, or ampicillin-sulbactam |
| Yes | Moxifloxacin, levofloxacin, or gemifloxacin | **or** one of these:<br>• Moxifloxacin<br>• Levofloxacin<br>• Gemifloxacin | **and**<br>• Moxifloxacin or levofloxacin<br><br>**and** possibly<br>• Vancomycin or linezolid for MRSA |

# Ventilator-Associated Pneumonia (VAP)

VAP is defined as a pneumonia developing more than 48 hours after intubation. The same features of severity apply as above. All are considered critical because the hypoxia is so severe that intubation was needed. VAP is treated more intensely than CAP because of the likelihood of resistant organisms. Use a combination of 3 drugs:

| ONE of these ... | ... and ONE of these ... | ... and ONE of these |
|---|---|---|
| Piperacillin-tazobactam, cefepime, or carbapenem (i.e., imipenem or meropenem) | Ciprofloxacin or levofloxacin | Vancomycin or linezolid |

Daptomycin is not usable for lung disease. Surfactant inactivates it.

# Pneumocystis Pneumonia (PCP)

Look for a person with HIV/AIDS and <200 CD4 cells/μL.

- Not taking PCP prophylaxis (bactrim [TMP/SMZ], dapsone, or atovaquone)
- Dry cough, dyspnea (particularly on exertion)
- Bilateral interstitial infiltrates
- Increased LDH
- Hypoxia on ABG

An ABG is particularly important in PCP because **steroids are added** if either:

- A-a gradient is >35
- $pO_2$ is <70 mmHg

It is very unlikely to have PCP with a normal LDH.

## Diagnostic Testing

When a person with AIDS, CD4 <200, and hypoxia has bilateral interstitial infiltrates, you still need to confirm that PCP is present.

- Bronchoscopy with bronchoalveolar lavage (BAL) is the standard of care
- Sputum stain is very specific if positive but can miss 50% of cases

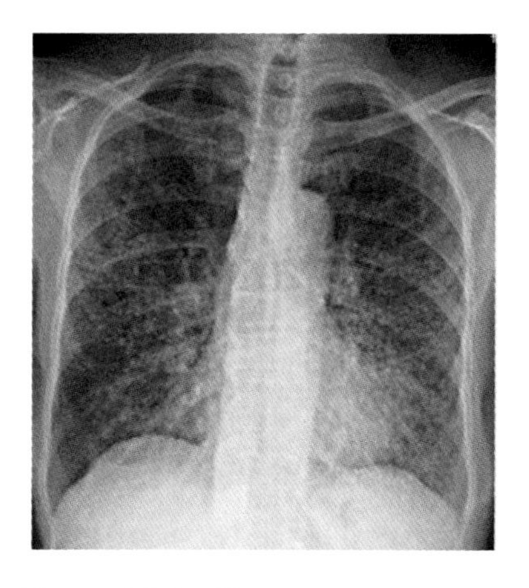

**Bilateral interstitial infiltrates as seen here can be from PCP, virus, mycoplasma, chlamydia, Coxiella pneumonia, or sarcoidosis.**

### Treatment

- Bactrim (TMP/SMZ): IV and oral therapy are nearly identical in efficacy
- Steroids if $pO_2$ <70 mmHg or A-a gradient >35
- Bactrim allergic patients: IV pentamidine, oral atovoquone, or clindamycin combined with primaquine

## Pleural Effusion

Pleural effusion is a collection of fluid inside the chest between the lung and chest wall. Pleural effusion can be caused by any of the following:

- Pneumonia
- Cancer
- Collagen-vascular (connective tissue) disorder (e.g., SLE)
- Trauma

Small effusions are asymptomatic. Large ones compress the lung and cause dyspnea.

## Diagnostic Testing

Confirm the presence of a pleural effusion with imaging studies. Fluid analysis is another important form of testing in effusion.

### Imaging Studies

The **lateral chest x-ray** is more sensitive than a posterior-anterior (PA) film for detecting pleural effusion.

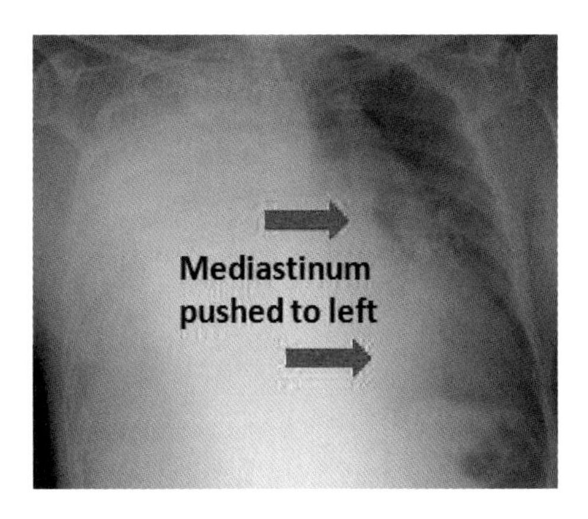


**Extremely large pleural effusion on the right pushing the mediastinum over to the left**

After the chest x-ray shows the effusion, the best next step is to do **decubitus films**—i.e., chest x-rays with the patient lying on one side. Most effusions "layer out," or move with gravity when the patient changes bodily position.

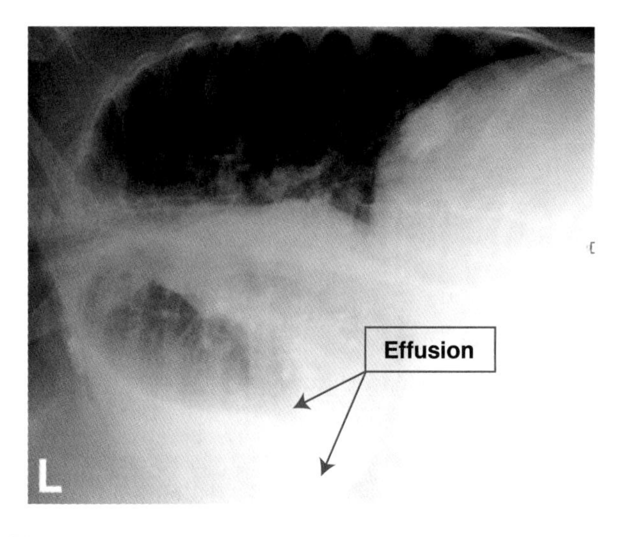


**Pleural fluid layers out as the patient lies on one side.**

If the presence of an effusion is unclear, there are 2 diagnostic options:

- **Chest CT scan**
- **Ultrasound** (U/S)

Sonographic (ultrasound) guidance helps in the detection of a loculated effusion, which does not move with a change in position. A loculated effusion is one that is walled off into smaller compartments by fibrous tissue.

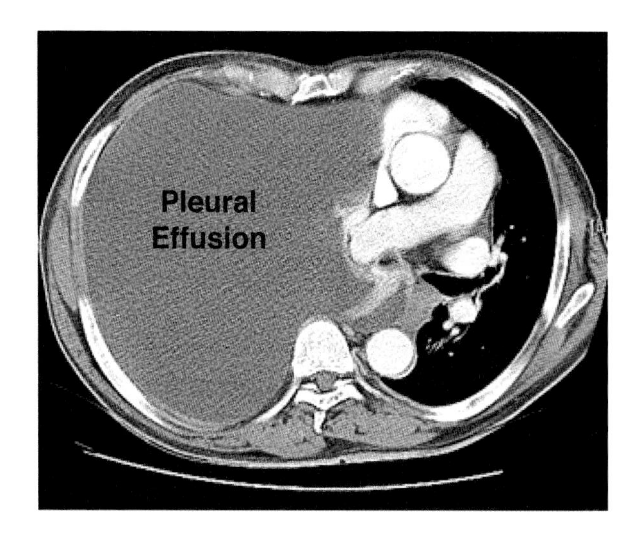


**Extremely large pleural effusion on the right pushing the mediastinum over to the left**

## Fluid Analysis

When there is a visible "layer" of fluid, you have a large effusion that should be examined for its content. The only way to do this is with a sample obtained by a needle via **thoracentesis**. In general, do thoracentesis for any effusion that forms a layer of 1 cm or more. Thoracentesis is often performed under sonographic guidance in order to prevent a pneumothorax from forming.

**Transudate:** lower level of protein and LDH

- CHF (Hydrostatic force in the heart)
- Hypoalbuminemia

**Exudate:** higher level of protein and LDH in effusion

- Cancer
- Infection
- Pulmonary embolus (PE)

- Connective tissue disease (e.g., SLE, Wegener's, rheumatoid arthritis)
- Pancreatic disease
- Lymphatic obstruction

| | Transudate | Exudate |
|---|---|---|
| **LDH** | <60% of serum | >60% of serum |
| **Protein** | <50% of serum | >50% of serum |

**Cell count:** Infection is associated with an effusion cell count >500–1,000, and usually higher. Bacterial infection should be predominantly neutrophils. Tuberculosis is predominantly lymphocytes. There is no single "cutoff" cell count that determines the presence or absence of infection.

**pH and glucose:** Infection lowers the pH and glucose level of pleural fluid. Infection eats glucose and makes acid. These and a high cell count in pleural fluid are the greatest indicators of the need for a chest tube to remove the fluid. pH ≤ 7.2 is a strong indicator of need for a chest tube.

**Round Saver**

Normal pleural pH is 7.6, not 7.4!

## Treatment

To clarify the significance of exudate vs. transudate, infected vs. noninfected, we must remember a few simple things. Chest tube drainage is performed under the following circumstances:

- **Definite:** infected (pH <7.2)
- **Possible:** cancer
- **Not performed:** uninfected transudate

| Pleural Fluid Analysis for Infection | |
|---|---|
| **Infection Unlikely** | **Infection Probable** |
| <500 WBCs | >500–1,000 WBCs |
| pH >7.3 | pH <7.2 |
| Drainage: no | Drainage: yes |

Normal fluid does not have eosinophils. Eosinophils in amounts >10% are from:

- Trauma
- Pneumothorax
- Cancer
- Drugs

## Pulmonary Embolism/ Thromboembolic Disease

Pulmonary embolism (PE) presents with shortness of breath that develops over a few minutes or a few hours. It can be so fast that patient is able to identify a very specific time when it started. Lung exam is normal. In PE there is no wheezing as in asthma, and no consolidation or dullness as in pneumonia or an effusion. In fact, wheezing and dullness strongly suggest a diagnosis other than PE.

- Tachycardia: extremely common
- Tachypnea
- Hemoptysis

**Sudden dyspnea + clear lung exam + x-ray normal = PE**

### Things You Will Be Asked on Rounds

- Any long plane rides this week?
- Any surgery in the last week or two?
- Possible injury to the leg?
- Cancer? (previous or current)

## Diagnostic Testing

| Test | Most Common Finding | Most Common Abnormality |
|---|---|---|
| Chest x-ray | Normal | Atelectasis |
| EKG | Sinus tachycardia | Nonspecific ST-T changes |
| ABG | Respiratory alkalosis | Low $pCO_2$, high pH |

Chest x-ray can sometimes show pleural effusion and pleural-based infection. EKG can sometimes show right axis deviation, right bundle branch block, and S1Q3T3.

Try to do the ABG on room air, because the A-a gradient is needed. A normal ABG does not absolutely exclude a PE.

### Round Saver

You will be asked about CXR, ABG, and EKG on all suspected PE patients.

The best confirmatory test to confirm PE is CT angiogram (CTA). Pulse oximetry is very misleading. Saturation >90% excludes nothing.

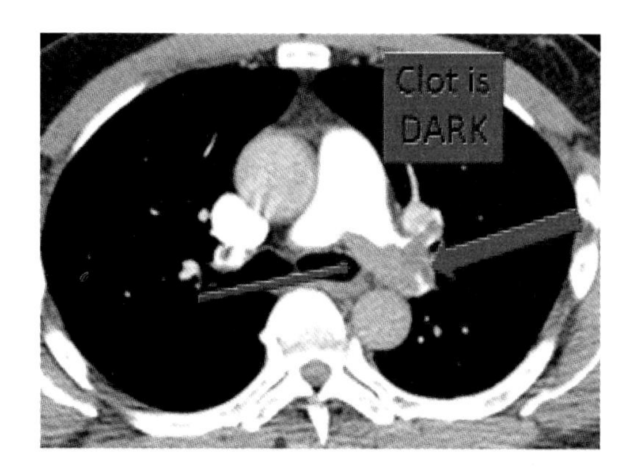


**Contrast material is white; it is blocked by the clot. Dark is abnormal.**

| Test | Pros | Cons |
|---|---|---|
| **CT angiogram (CTA)** | 98% sensitive/ specific for large clots | • Needs IV contrast<br>• Varies with reader skill<br>• May miss small peripheral clots |
| **D-dimer** | >95% sensitive | • Nonspecific; bleeding or clotting anywhere makes it (+)<br>• Cannot detect recurrences |
| **Leg duplex** | Positive test eliminates need for any other test | • Misses 1/3 of clots that may have embolized or are from pelvic veins |
| **V/Q scan** | • No contrast = no nephrotoxicity<br>• Completely normal perfusion scan excludes clots | • Much less precise than CTA<br>• Low probability scan misses 15%<br>• High probability scan false (+) rate is 15% |
| **Pulmonary angiography** | Most accurate of all tests | • Needs catheter insertion into right heart<br>• 2% mortality |

With echocardiography:

- Assesses right ventricular "strain"
- Pulmonary hypertension
- Tricuspid regurgitation
- Helps find large clots that need thrombolytics
- Misses most smaller clots

## Treatment

Do not wait for the CT angiogram to give oxygen and heparin. ABG (hypoxia, low $pCO_2$) and risks such as immobility, cancer, surgery, or trauma really help determine who needs heparin immediately.

- Start warfarin at same time as heparin
- Unstable (SBP <90) means consider thrombolytics
- Can't anticoagulate: place vena cava filter

Once the chest x-ray, EKG, and ABG are done and suggest PE:

- Start heparin: low molecular weight (LMW) is as good as or better than IV heparin
- Evaluate unstable patients for thrombolytics
- Start warfarin right away with the heparin: plan for 6 months of therapy
- If you can't anticoagulate, place an inferior vena cava (IVC) filter

If the PE recurs while on heparin, place an IVC filter.

For the largest clots, which result in hemodynamic instability, thrombolytics are used. Look for:

- Hypotension (SBP <90 mmHg) with tachycardia
- Persistent hypoxia despite high-flow oxygen use
- Echo with pulmonary hypertension, right ventricular (RV) hypertrophy, and tricuspid regurgitation

Consider using a catheter to remove clots when thrombolytics cannot be given or fail:

- Used when massive clots produce instability
- Used when IVC filter has not been effective
- Alternative to surgical embolectomy

With warfarin use, start warfarin at the same time as heparin.

- Do not worry about "warfarin-induced skin necrosis," as the person is already on heparin
- Need 2–3 days minimum to see an effect
- INR 2–3 is the goal
- Plan 6 months of therapy

**Round Saver**

Does the patient have a doctor? Who will check the INR after discharge?

In patients with no identifiable risk factor such as trauma, immobility, cancer, or surgery, you will need to think about why a clot occurred. Possibilities:

- Factor V Leiden mutation (most common)
- Anti-phospholipid syndrome (APS) (most likely to recur)
- Deficiency of protein C, protein S, and antithrombin

Evaluation for most causes of thrombophilia cannot occur during the acute clot, as heparin and warfarin use render the tests inaccurate. The only cause that makes a difference in treatment with the first clot is APS. APS has such a high risk of recurrence that you might begin lifelong treatment with warfarin after only one clot. Just remember, warfarin causes bleeding.

# ASTHMA

## Acute Asthma Exacerbation

Look for a patient with:

- Sudden onset of dyspnea
- Wheezing on examination
- Most patients have a previous history of asthma

Infection, cold weather, and not taking medications can cause asthma exacerbation.

How can you tell whether an acute exacerbation is severe?

- Fast respiratory rate (>30/min)
- Low peak flow (<100–200)
- Respiratory acidosis

You must try to find out why the patient is having this episode. Most patients will have an identifiable cause, such as infection or not taking their medications. This is critical to know, because if there is no identifiable cause of the exacerbation, it means the patient will need more medication added to the treatment plan long term.

### Things You Will Be Asked on Rounds

**Acute Asthma Exacerbation—Tracking the Cause**

- Presence of fever?
- Actual temperature reading, or just feeling of warmth?
- Medication routine: consistent or inconsistent?
- Health insurance to cover medications?
- Loss of job/loss of insurance?
- Occurrence of this episode after exercise?
- Emotional event before this episode?
- New animal in the house or construction?

## Diagnostic Testing

Prior to initiating therapy, only the peak flow needs to be done: a single hard "blow" through a tube that measures the "peak flow." The results are closest to an FEV1 in terms of meaning. There is no "normal" peak flow, since it is based on the person's height.

> **Round Saver**
> Ask patients if they know their usual peak flow.

Other tests to routinely get in an asthma exacerbation are:

- Chest x-ray:
  - Look for pneumonia
  - Normal x-ray does not exclude infection as the cause of the asthma exacerbation
  - Fever + a new infiltrate = treat CAP
- ABG:
  - Get ABG if dyspnea is severe; not clearly needed in all cases
  - Routine exacerbation shows a respiratory alkalosis (low $pCO_2$)
  - Respiratory acidosis (low pH, high $pCO_2$) needs the ICU and possible intubation

In acute asthma, hurry up the treatment. Use albuterol, steroids, and ipratropium right away.

## Treatment

For **acute cases** of asthma exacerbation, use albuterol inhalers. There is no maximum dose in acute asthma.

- Glucocorticoids
- Ipratropium helps in the emergency department
- Magnesium may be helpful

| Medications for Acute Asthma Treatment | | |
|---|---|---|
| **Medication Class** | **Individual Drug Names** | **Key Points** |
| Beta-2 agonists | Albuterol<br>Levalbuterol<br>Pirbuterol | • Severely ill patients can get one right after the other<br>• No maximum dose<br>• Levalbuterol is not better than albuterol |
| Glucocorticoids | Prednisone<br>Methylprednisolone | • Not clear that IV treatment is better than oral if patient can take pills<br>• Steroids need 4–6 hours to work, *so order them fast* |
| Anticholinergics | Ipratropium | • Ipratropium is given in 3 doses 20 minutes apart<br>• Tiotropium is not used for acute exacerbation |

Medications that **do not help** acute exacerbations are as follows:

- Theophylline, aminophylline
- Montelukast, zafirlukast
- Cromolyn, nedocromil

**Round Saver** 

If your attending "believes in" levalbuterol, it is a religious conviction, not a medical fact.

### How NOT to Kill Your Patient

- Albuterol has no maximum dose if the patient can't breathe.
- Don't wait for tests if the patient is dyspneic and wheezing—treat now!
- Steroids need 4–6 hours to start to working, so hurry up!
- Find the cause of the exacerbation.
- Respiratory acidosis in acute asthma needs an ICU evaluation.
- If the patient uses inhaled steroids, do not stop use during the acute exacerbation. They need 5–10 days to reach a maximum effect.

## When Can the Patient Be Discharged?

- They simply "feel" better
- Respiratory rate normalizes
- Peak flow increases
- Wheezing improves: it does not have to be entirely gone

## Discharge Medications

- Restart usual home/outpatient medications
- Oral steroids for 5–10 days
- Consider adding a new chronic "controller medication"
- Do **not** wait for oral steroids to be finished to start inhaled steroids. Inhaled steroids take 5–10 days to reach a maximum effect

## Acute Asthma Diagnosis Is Not Clear

When patients are admitted with acute dyspnea, it is often unclear whether asthma or "reactive airways" are the cause. You may not always clearly hear wheezing on examination.

### Round Saver

BNP is up in CHF.

- Pre- and post-bronchodilation pulmonary function testing (PFTs) can be part of this evaluation
- Look for **12% increase in forced expiratory volume** in one second (FEV1) after the use of albuterol

## Office or Clinic Asthma Management

### Establishing the Diagnosis

When patients present with dyspnea and clear wheezing, the diagnosis is straightforward. When wheezing is absent at the time of the office visit, pulmonary function testing (PFT) can be useful to establish the diagnosis. Asthma can show:

- Decrease in FEV1
- Decrease in FEV1 ratio to forced vital capacity (FVC)

If there is no wheezing and the FEV1/FVC is normal, the single most specific test is bronchoprovocation. Bronchoprovocation means measuring the FEV1 after inhaling methacholine. If there are reactive airways, the FEV1 will decrease by 20%.

## Treatment

The best initial therapy for asthma is as-needed use of an inhaled beta agonist such as albuterol. If the patient is still dyspneic, then add an inhaled glucocorticoid such as fluticasone, budesonide, beclomethasone, or mometasone. All inhaled steroids are equal in efficacy.

The next step is to add an inhaled long-acting beta agonist (LABA) such as salmeterol or formoterol.

If the combination of inhaled steroid + albuterol as needed + LABA is not effective, the best next treatment to add is not entirely clear. This is when treatment becomes a matter of trying different therapies and looking for a clinical response. Options are:

- Leukotriene inhibitor (montelukast, zafirlukast)
- Theophylline
- Mast cell stabilizers (cromolyn, nedocromil)

Omalizumab is an anti-IgE antibody that is used in those who have severe asthma not controlled with the other medications. It is used as one of the last steps to keep the patient off long-term oral steroids.

The last thing to try is chronic oral glucocorticoids such as prednisone. The problem with chronic prednisone use is adverse effects.

### Adverse Effects of Glucocorticoids

- Osteoporosis
- Abnormal fat distribution such as facial rounding
- Male-pattern hair loss
- Skin thinning, bruising
- Acne
- Hyperlipidemia, hyperglycemia
- Cataracts

### Asthma Treatment Summary

1. Albuterol as needed to start
2. Add inhaled glucocorticoids
3. Add long-acting beta agonist (LABA)
4. Add montelukast
5. Add theophylline, cromolyn, or omalizumab on a case-by-case basis
6. Systemic glucocorticoids

## Chronic Obstructive Pulmonary Disease (COPD)

COPD is managed in much the same way as asthma, except that there is much less response. Only half of patients with COPD will have a meaningful response to inhaled bronchodilators such as albuterol. The only test to confirm significant "reactive airways" is PFTs. As when establishing a diagnosis of asthma, look for a 12% increase in FEV1 after the use of albuterol.

> **Round Saver**
>
> PFTs cannot be done during an acute dyspneic episode.

### Diagnostic Testing

1. ABG is critical in acute exacerbation of COPD:
   - ABG is the only way to tell if there is significant $CO_2$ retention or decrease in pH.
   - ABG indicates the need for intubation.
   - Severe respiratory acidosis needs ICU evaluation.
2. Chest x-ray on all patients

## Treatment

Round Saver

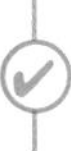

Give just enough oxygen to get the saturation to 90%.

Treat acute exacerbation of COPD with:

1. Albuterol (same as in asthma; no limit on frequency of treatment)
2. Systemic glucocorticoids such as prednisone
3. Ipratropium
4. Antibiotics if there is increased sputum production and purulence even without fever or a new abnormality on chest x-ray
5. Try CPAP or BiPAP (noninvasive ventilation) before you intubate a severely ill COPD patient.

### Antibiotic Use in Acute Exacerbation of COPD (AECOPD)

Use of antibiotics is more liberal in COPD than in an exacerbation of asthma. In asthma you should use antibiotics only if there is definite evidence of lung infection such as a fever, leukocytosis, and infiltrate on chest x-ray. In COPD, antibiotics are indicated for increasing dyspnea with:

- Increased sputum volume
- Increased sputum purulence

For **uncomplicated AECOPD** (<65, infrequent hospitalizations, no recent antibiotics, no heart disease), choose any *one* of the following:

- Macrolide (azithromycin, clarithromycin)
- Doxycycline
- Cefuroxime, cefpodoxime, cefdinir
- TMP/SMZ

For **complicated AECOPD** (>65, frequent hospitalizations, antibiotic use, heart disease present), choose:

- Moxifloxacin, levofloxacin, gemifloxacin

## Management Differences between COPD and Asthma in COPD

- Tiotropium and ipratropium are as good as albuterol
- Supplemental oxygen lowers mortality if $pO_2$ <60 mmHg (saturation <90%) on room air
- Absolute indispensability of smoking cessation
- Leukotriene inhibitors (e.g., montelukast) do not help
- Mast cell stabilizers (e.g., cromolyn) and magnesium do not help

## Outpatient Management of COPD

### Establishing the Diagnosis

PFTs in COPD will show:

- Both decreased FEV1 and decreased FVC
- FEV1 decreased more than FVC (decreased ratio)
- Increased total lung capacity
- Increased residual volume

Chest x-ray will show:

- Hyperinflation
- Flattened diaphragm
- Bullae possible

### Outpatient Treatment of COPD

1. Albuterol as needed to start
2. Add tiotropium (superior to ipratropium)
3. Add inhaled glucocorticoids
4. Add LABA such as salmeterol or formoterol
5. Oxygen for hypoxic patients ($pO_2$ <60 mmHg or saturation <90% on room air)

**Round Saver**

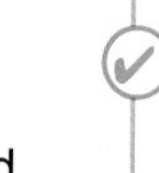

LABAs such as salmeterol should never be used as a single agent

6. Pneumococcal and influenza vaccination
7. Smoking cessation is absolutely critical

COPD patients who have reactive airways or bronchospasm found on PFTs have more therapeutic options. If a patient really has only COPD as emphysema, there is not much you can do for them except make sure they stop smoking and use oxygen at home when they develop severe hypoxia.

## Tuberculosis (TB)

Like pneumonia, TB presents with fever, cough, sputum production, and possibly dyspnea. The main differences between the presentation of TB and pneumonia are:

- Chronicity: often symptomatic for weeks to months
- Weight loss
- Origin: two thirds occur in recent immigrants from developing countries
- Social factors: injection drug users, incarcerated patients, homeless shelter dwellers

### Diagnostic Testing

- Chest x-ray
- 3 sputum acid fast stains for TB

**Round Saver**

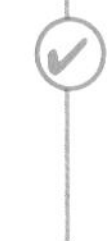

Risk factors for exposure matter more in TB than in any other lung infection.

### Treatment

Remember to place the patient on respiratory isolation while evaluating for TB.

Before starting treatment for TB, obtain 3 sputum samples for acid-fast bacilli (AFB). It is far preferable to await results of the stain because treatment will decrease the yield of AFB culture even if used only for a few days. You do not have to wait for results of culture if the AFB stain is positive. Except in certain areas with a high immigrant population, TB is uncommon.

If **any** of the AFB stains is positive, start 4 anti-TB drugs: rifampin, isoniazid, pyrazinamide, and ethambutol. All 4 TB drugs can cause liver toxicity. Do not stop the medications unless the AST and ALT have risen to 3–5 times the upper limit of normal.

**Round Saver**

All first-line TB meds cause liver toxicity.

| TB Medications | |
|---|---|
| **Drug** | **Adverse Effects** |
| Rifampin | Red/orange body fluids |
| Isoniazid | Neuropathy, vitamin B6 deficiency |
| Pyrazinamide | Hyperuricemia (do not treat) |
| Ethambutal | Optic neuritis (color vision first) |

### Duration of Therapy

The standard duration for treating pulmonary TB is 6 months. All 4 drugs are used for the first 2 months. After 2 months, if the organism is fully sensitive, you stop ethambutal and pyrazinamide and continue isoniazid and rifampin for 4 more months, for a total of 6 months.

**Exceptions.** The total duration of TB treatment exceeds 6 months for:

- Osteomyelitis
- Meningitis
- Miliary TB
- Pregnancy

**Round Saver**

No pyrazinamide in pregnancy.

Of these, only pregnancy has a clear duration of treatment, which is 9 months. The others get 9–18 months of treatment, depending on the site and the sensitivity of the organism.

| TB Therapy | | | |
|---|---|---|---|
| **Months 1–2**<br>• Rifampin<br>• Isoniazid<br>• Pyrazinamide<br>• Ethambutal | **Months 3–18**<br>• Rifampin<br>• Isoniazid | | |
| | **Months 3–6** | **Months 7–9** | **Months 10–18** |
| Pulmonary | yes | | |
| Pregnancy | yes | yes | |
| Bone, CNS, miliary | yes | yes | yes (duration depends on site & sensitivity of organism) |

## Management of Latent TB

In the United States, screening for latent TB is only given to those at high risk. Neither the PPD nor the interferon-gamma release assay (IGRA) is a screening test for the general public. The IGRA is a lab test that is done on freshly processed lymphocytes. The IGRA has the same meaning as the PPD skin test, except that it does not cross-react with BCG, the TB vaccine used outside the United States.

**Round Saver**

Anyone getting isoniazid needs vitamin $B_6$.

### Who to Screen?

Groups at high risk, such as:

- Recent (<5 years) immigrants from developing countries
- Healthcare workers
- Prisoners
- Alcoholics
- Chronic prednisone users (>15 mg/day)
- Close contacts of those with TB
- HIV-positive persons

### PPD Testing

The PPD should not be done as an in-hospital test on patients with acute, symptomatic respiratory illness. Rather, symptomatic patients with cough, sputum, and abnormal chest x-rays need their sputum tested by AFB stain.

> **Round Saver**
>
> Prepare your mind to see *many* people use the PPD inappropriately!

Only induration (raised skin) indicates a positive PPD test. Redness does not count.

> **Round Saver**
>
> The #1 incorrect use of IGRA/PPD is in acutely ill patients.

| Induration Size | Indicates Positive Latent TB Result For | Notes |
|---|---|---|
| 5 mm | • HIV positive persons<br>• Chronic prednisone (steroid) users<br>• Patients whose abnormal x-rays are consistent with old granulomas<br>• Close contacts of those with TB (does not include health-care workers) | "Close contact" for purposes of the PPD test means exposure 4–6 hours a day for minimum 1–2 weeks. |
| 10 mm | • HIV positive<br>• Chronic prednisone (steroid) use<br>• Abnormal x-rays consistent with old granulomas | |
| 15 mm | • Persons with no risks | Confusing, because people with no risks should never have been tested at all! |

Some people need **two-stage PPD testing** (i.e., 2 PPD tests to exclude previous exposure):

- Persons never PPD tested before
- Those with no PPD within the last 2 years

A second PPD test is done when the first test might be falsely negative because the person was exposed a long time ago. It is done 1–2 weeks later. If negative, the second test confirms that there is no latent TB. If reactive, it is a true positive.

### Interferon-Gamma Release Assay (IGRA)

- Same sensitivity as a PPD
- No cross-reaction with BCG
- A blood test on fresh lymphocytes; delay in processing ruins the test

### Treatment of Latent TB

Both a positive PPD and IGRA are treated with isoniazid (INH) for 9 months. All patients getting isoniazid anytime need supplemental pyridoxine (vitamin B6).

> **Round Saver**
> Only 10% with positive PPD or IGRA ever develop TB.

- Get a chest x-ray *before* INH is started
- If the x-ray has an abnormality, check sputum to exclude active disease
- If the x-ray is normal, give INH for 9 months
- Do not repeat the PPD in the future. It will always be reactive.

> **Round Saver**
> Everyone with a positive PPD or IGRA needs a chest x-ray.

## Allergic Bronchopulmonary Aspergillosis (ABPA)

Some patients with asthma, cystic fibrosis, or bronchiectasis become colonized with aspergillosis. This is, by definition, not an invasive aspergillosis. It is like "contact dermatitis" of the bronchi to aspergillus antigens. That is why the mainstay of treatment is oral steroids, not antifungals.

Look for:

- Intermittent and repeated episodes of dyspnea in asthmatics
- "Brownish" flecks or plugs in sputum
- Fleeting (migrating) infiltrates on chest x-ray that appear at different sites
- Increased eosinophil count on complete blood count (CBC)

## Diagnostic Testing

ABPA has no single "gold standard" test. You will use a combination of:

- Infiltrates/central bronchiectasis on chest CT
- Skin test reactivity to aspergillus
- High IgE levels in blood
- Blood "precipitating antibodies" to aspergillus

## Treatment

1. Oral glucocorticoids such as prednisone for at least 2 weeks and as long as 3–6 months
2. Antifungals: For recurrences or steroid unresponsive patients. Use oral itraconazole or voriconazole.

**Round Saver**

Inhaled steroids do not work for ABPA.

## Solitary Pulmonary Nodule

Lesions suggestive of possible malignancy need biopsy. Benign lesions should be followed with a repeat chest x-ray in 3–6 months.

| Benign | Malignant |
|---|---|
| Stable size | Growing |
| Small (<1 cm) | Large (>1–2 cm) |
| Nonsmoker | Smoker |
| Age <35 | Age >50 |
| Smooth, calcified | Irregular, spicules |

The type of biopsy needed depends on location. Use bronchoscopy to biopsy central lesions. Peripheral lesions are sampled with:

- CT-guided transthoracic biopsy
- Video-assisted thoracoscopy (VATS): this is putting a scope directly into the thoracic cavity
- Open lung or excisional biopsy: removes the whole lesion

## Bronchiectasis

- Recurrent episodes of lung infection
- Drainage and expectoration of large volumes of sputum by the cupful
- Higher volume than bronchitis
- Recurs more often than pneumonia
- Not collected into a walled-off area like an abscess
- Happens in those with long-term deformity of bronchi, such as from cystic fibrosis
- Chest CT is the most accurate test

- Treat infections as they arise
- No cure

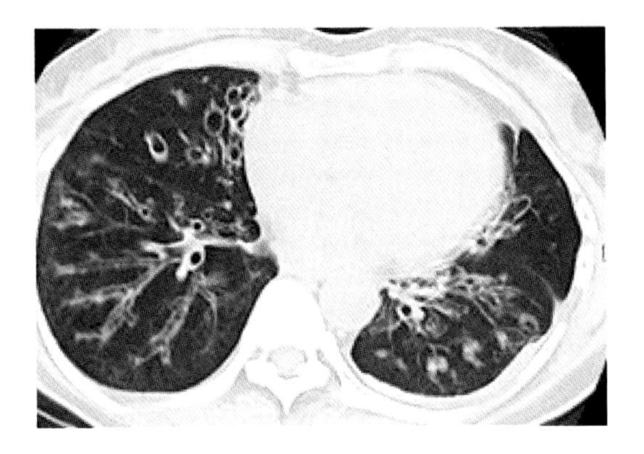

**Wide bronchi with very thick walls, sometimes called "tram-track" because of the abnormally increased width**

## Interstitial Lung Disease (ILD)

Interstitial lung disease (ILD) presents with:

- Chronic, slowly progressive shortness of breath
- Dry, nonproductive cough
- Rales "like velcro" on examination
- Clubbing is uncommon

### Etiology

ILD is a chronic fibrosis of the lungs that can be idiopathic, caused by previous exposure to inhaled irritants, or from medication. You cannot distinguish these by any aspect of the physical examination or chest x-ray. You can only distinguish them if you ask the patient about the exposure in the past.

- Asbestosis
- Coal dust

- Pneumoconiosis
- Mercury vapor from industry
- Cotton fibers (byssinosis)
- Berylliosis
- Medications: bleomycin, nitrofurantoin
- Connective tissue diseases: scleroderma, rheumatoid arthritis, sarcoidosis

## Diagnostic Testing

- Chest x-ray:
    - Bilateral disease
    - Interstitial or reticulonodular when more chronic and severe
    - Effusion is rare
    - Focal infiltrates occur because of recurrent pneumonia
- Chest CT: same as the x-ray but with more detail
- PFTs: restrictive lung disease
    - Decrease in all lung volumes
    - Decrease in both FEV1 and FVC but the decrease is proportionate
    - Decrease in diffusion capacity of carbon monoxide (DLCO)
- Biopsy: most accurate (and most invasive) test
- Echocardiogram:
    - Right ventricular (RV) hypertrophy
    - Tricuspid regurgitation (pulmonary hypertension)

## Treatment

There is very little disease-specific therapy. Steroids are useful in sarcoidosis and some connective tissue diseases, and they are tried in idiopathic disease for a short time. Scleroderma is given a trial of cyclophosphamide.

## Pulmonary Hypertension

All forms of ILD can lead to pulmonary hypertension. Separate from these diseases, a small number of patients have a "primary" pulmonary hypertension—basically a tightening of the pulmonary artery without identifiable lung fibrosis or hypoxia. If a patient has pulmonary hypertension from hypoxia, such as in COPD, it is not "primary" pulmonary hypertension. In those cases the management is to correct the underlying cause.

In primary pulmonary hypertension:

- The lungs themselves are normal
- Chest x-ray and chest CT show normal air space
- Echocardiogram is the mainstay of diagnosis
- Right heart catheterization is the most accurate test

### Treatment

Chronic home oxygen is used to keep the oxygen saturation >90% and the $pO_2$ >60 mmHg.

Specific therapy includes:

- Bosentan (endothelin antagonist)
- Treprostinil, iloprost (prostacyclin inhibitors)
- Calcium channel blockers
- Sildenafil

**Round Saver**

Primary pulmonary hypertension treatment is beyond the scope of a generalist. Consultation is critical.

# Obstructive Sleep Apnea (OSA)

OSA presents with:

- Daytime somnolence/poor concentration
- Obesity with a short fat neck
- Snoring reported by sleep partner
- Hypertension and erectile dysfunction for unclear reasons

> **Round Saver**
>
> 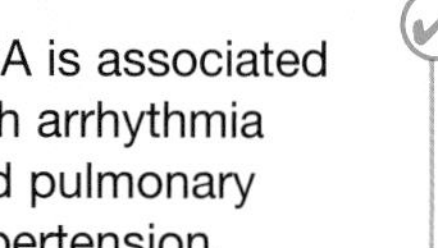
>
> OSA is associated with arrhythmia and pulmonary hypertension.

Risk factors include:

- Hypothyroidism
- Acromegaly (surrounding neck tissues grow)

## Diagnostic Testing

- Polysomnography (sleep study)
- Multiple (>5/hour) periods of apnea/hypopnea (severe disease >30/hour)

## Treatment

1. Lifestyle modifications
   - Weight loss
   - Exercise
   - Sleep on your side
   - Decrease alcohol

> **Round Saver**
>
> 
>
> There is no clearly effective drug therapy for OSA.

2. Oral appliances: worn to protrude the jaw forward during sleep
3. Positive airway pressure
   - Continuous positive airway pressure (CPAP)
   - Bilevel positive airway pressure (BiPAP)
4. Surgical correction of the narrowed airway

# Acute Respiratory Distress Syndrome (ARDS)

ARDS is diffuse lung injury of unclear etiology. The chest x-ray looks like pulmonary edema is present but the echocardiogram and (when done) right heart catheter show normal lung and pulmonary artery pressures.

Sepsis, burns, aspiration of gastric contents, pancreatitis, and a number of acute, severe systemic illnesses are associated with ARDS, but the precise cause is simply unknown.

ARDS presentation involves:

- Tachypnea, tachycardia, and rales on examination
- Possible fever and hypotension from the precipitating cause of the ARDS
- Usually a person on a ventilator

## Diagnostic Testing

There is no test to prove someone has ARDS. It is simply defined as:

- Acute, severe lung injury
- Absence of pulmonary edema with normal vascular pressures (wedge $<18$ mmHg)

Evaluate for ARDS using the **$PaO_2/FiO_2$ ratio:**

- $FiO_2$ is blood oxygenation level in mmHg. Normal $PaO_2 =$ 100 mmHg.
- Fraction of inspired oxygen ($FiO_2$) is expressed as a decimal. For instance:
    - 20% oxygen on room air is 0.2
    - 50% oxygen by face mask is 0.5
- $PaO_2/FiO_2 <300$ = acute lung injury (ALI).
- $PaO_2/FiO_2 <200$ = ARDS.

So, if you have a $pO_2$ of 100 mmHg while breathing room air (0.2), your ratio ($PaO_2/FiO_2$) = 500. If you have $pO_2$ of 60 mmHg while breathing 30% oxygen, your ratio = 60/0.3 = 200, i.e., diagnosis of ARDS.

### Treatment

- Nothing reverses ARDS.
- Sedate, support, oxygenate, and . . . wait!

## Sarcoidosis

**Asymptomatic** sarcoidosis can present as an incidental finding of bilateral hilar adenopathy on a chest x-ray. The most accurate test is a biopsy of the nodes showing noncaseating granulomas. If there are no symptoms, no treatment is needed.

Sarcoidosis, when **symptomatic,** presents as:

- Dyspnea worsened with exertion
- Dry cough
- No fever

Uncommon extrapulmonary manifestations include:

- Skin: the most common site outside the lung
- Neurological: facial nerve palsy can be bilateral; stroke is rare
- Cardiac: AV block, restrictive cardiomyopathy
- Renal, liver, and spleen: involvement is common on autopsy but clinically silent

## Diagnostic Testing

- Chest x-ray shows hilar adenopathy in 95% of patients. Lung fibrosis is less common.
- Hypercalcemia 10%
- ACE level elevation 60%
- EKG with conduction defect <5%
- Noncaseating granuloma on biopsy is essential to establish the diagnosis

**Round Saver**

No blood test diagnoses sarcoidosis. ACE levels are clinically useless.

## Treatment

Prednisone is effective in nearly all patients

# Lung Abscess

Normal people do not get a lung abscess. Look for:

- High volume aspiration + bad teeth + bad smell
- Chronicity, weight loss, and fever

To get a lung abscess, you must lose your gag reflex for at least a short time. Look for:

- Stroke
- Seizure
- Intubation
- Alcoholism/intoxication

Lung abscess begins with aspiration that causes chemical burn or pneumonitis. Pneumonia/infection develops next, and then cavitation takes several weeks. Lung abscess is very rare. It occurs only in a person who avoids care such as antibiotics for several weeks.

## Diagnostic Testing

1. Chest x-ray first to show a cavity
2. Chest CT shows cavity in greater detail
3. Biopsy for a specific culture

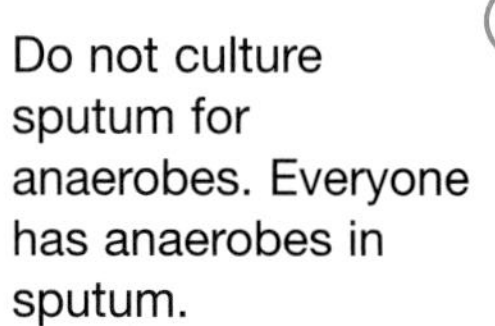

**Round Saver**

Do not culture sputum for anaerobes. Everyone has anaerobes in sputum.

## Treatment

Cover oral anaerobes:

- Clindamycin
- Ampicillin-sulbactam (Unasyn)
- Piperacillin-tazobactam (Zosyn)

**Round Saver**

Metronidazole alone is insufficient for lung abscess. Metronidazole covers GI anaerobes.

# Rheumatology 10

Rheumatologic diseases are treated most often in the outpatient setting. However, since they may be in the past medical history of a given inpatient, their understanding is important.

The disorders in this chapter are presented in the order of frequency in which they are most likely to be seen on your first rotation.

## Septic Arthritis

An infected joint presents with monoarticular arthritis usually of a single large joint such as the knee. Look for:

- Redness
- Warmth
- Immobility
- Swelling
- Fever

Unless there is a clear history of gout, there is no way to be sure if the joint is inflamed with infection or inflammation such as gout before doing the arthrocentesis.

### Things You Will Be Asked on Rounds

Find out initially:

- Presence of fever?
- If joint is hot, red, swollen, tender, immobile
- Blood WBC count
- PT/INR and platelet count (but then say, "They don't matter, tap the joint anyway")
- Synovial fluid cell count, stain and crystal analysis (must know)
- Percentage of neutrophils (differential) on the fluid (must know)
- Was first dose of vancomycin and ceftriaxone actually given?

Radiologic tests do not exclude anything. The more abnormal a joint is, the more likely there is to be an infection.

### Things You Will Be Asked on Rounds

If there are abnormal joints, find out:

- Prior joint disease
- Osteoarthritis
- Rheumatoid arthritis
- Joint replacement
- Sexual history (though extremely unreliable)

### Round Saver

Any cause of bacteremia can seed the joint.

## Diagnostic Testing

> **Round Saver**
> Tap the joint **before** giving antibiotics.

There is no noninvasive way to establish a diagnosis of septic arthritis. Potentially infected joints can be diagnosed only with arthrocentesis (joint tap). Leukocytosis and blood cultures are suggestive of septic or infectious arthritis but are not conclusive. Imaging studies (x-ray, CT, MRI, etc.) do not help diagnose joint infection.

There is no need to wait for coagulation testing or platelet count prior to tapping the joint. That is because the likelihood of bleeding into a joint is extremely low.

### Synovial Fluid Analysis

| Test | • Septic arthritis<br>• Staph/Strep | • Septic arthritis<br>• Gonorrhea | Gout | Pseudogout (CPPD disease) |
|---|---|---|---|---|
| Cell count | >50,000 WBCs | 20,000–50,000 WBCs | 10,000–20,000 WBCs | 10,000–20,000 WBCs |
| Differential | >80–90% PMNs | >80–90% PMNs | 50:50 PMNs | 50:50 PMNs |
| Gram stain | 50–60% | <25% | N/A | N/A |
| Blood culture | 25–50% | 10% | N/A | N/A |
| Specific test | Joint fluid culture<br>90% sensitive | Joint fluid 50%<br>Combination of sites AND joint fluid 90% | Crystals<br>Negative birefringent needles | Crystals<br>Positive birefringent rhomboids |

CPPD = calcium pyrophosphate deposition disease; PMN = polymorphonuclear cells (neutrophil); N/A = not applicable

### Confirmatory Testing of Septic Arthritis

Look for increased synovial fluid WBC count >50,000–100,000. Occasionally patients may have lower cell counts, initially confusing diagnosis with gout or CPPD disease (pseudogout). Confirm with:

- Synovial fluid Gram stain
- Synovial fluid culture

**Round Saver**

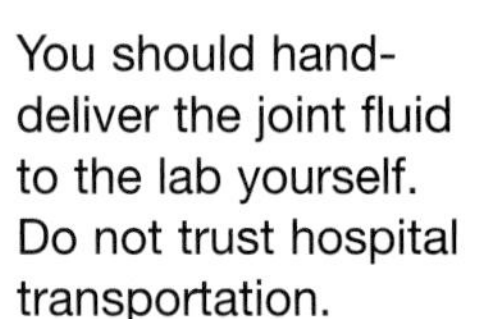

You should hand-deliver the joint fluid to the lab yourself. Do not trust hospital transportation.

**Round Saver**

Do not wait! Call or go to the lab to get Gram-stain results.

### Confirmatory Testing of Disseminated Gonorrhea

The *Gonococcus* is extremely difficult to grow from disseminated sites. In addition to joint fluid, the following sites must all be cultured:

- Cervix
- Urethra
- Pharynx
- Rectum
- Blood

Remember to culture the blood at least **twice** prior to starting antibiotics.

## Treatment

If the synovial fluid cell count comes back with >10,000–20,000 WBCs, start **both**:

- Vancomycin 1 gram q12 hours IV **and**
- Ceftriaxone 1 gram q24 hours IV

Although septic arthritis usually has >50,000 WBC/mcL, even a moderate elevation in WBC means you should start antibiotics. Stop them if the joint fluid culture is negative 48–72 hours later.

- The first doses of all antibiotics should be given **stat** (urgently).
- You do not need to inject antibiotics directly into a joint.
- Clearly septic joints (>50,000 WBC/mcL) need orthopedic referral to wash them out.
- Cell counts in the middle (20,000–30,000 WBC/mcL) are confusing.
- "No growth" on synovial fluid:
    - excludes septic arthritis with *Staphylococcus, Streptococcus,* and Gram-negative bacilli.
    - **does not exclude gonorrhea**.
- Any bacteremia seeds the joints.
- When in doubt, treat both infections and gout.

**Round Saver** 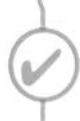

Confirm that your antibiotics have been given, not just ordered.

Ceftriaxone is safe if the penicillin allergy is only a rash.

## Osteomyelitis

On the medical service, almost all osteomyelitis is caused by diabetes and peripheral vascular disease. *Make sure you ask.* Trauma should not be on the medical service.

Look for an ulcer in a diabetic patient with redness, warmth, and swelling. Tenderness is not conclusive. Diabetics have neuropathy that makes bad infections painless. A bad ulcer with no pain is serious. There may be drainage of pus (purulent material) from the ulcer.

**Round Saver** 

Most common osteomyelitis mistakes:

- Culturing the surface of an ulcer
- Swabbing draining sinus tract

## Diagnostic Testing

- Do an x-ray first.
  - If the x-ray is normal: do an MRI.
  - If the x-ray shows osteomyelitis: no MRI needed.
- ESR or C-reactive protein (CRP):
  - Normal excludes osteomyelitis
  - Abnormal is used to follow response to treatment
- If the x-ray or MRI shows osteomyelitis, have a bone biopsy done **before** starting antibiotics.

**Bone biopsy** is indispensable in treating bone infection:

- It tells you what organism is in the bone; x-ray, MRI, and bone scan cannot.
- It tells you what the organism is to; x-ray, MRI, and bone scan cannot.
- A swab culture of ulcer is worse than useless; it distracts you from the real organism.

Do a biopsy before giving antibiotics:

- If antibiotics are given for 1–2 days before a biopsy is done, you decrease the yield of the culture.
- If you treat a sensitive *Staphylococcus* with vancomycin, there is far greater failure than if you use cephalosporin or penicillin.

Osteomyelitis is not an emergency, so waiting an extra day is not a problem.

Expect that people will misunderstand the diagnostic tests for osteomyelitis. You are on your first medicine rotation, so remember that you can't just make a statement. You need to show proof to your attending or resident about why he or she is wrong.

**Round Saver** 

Do not disagree with the residents or attending in front of others. Do show proof and evidence.

Blood cultures positive in 10% of patients can spare the need for bone biopsy.

The **nuclear bone scan** is not specific. It should be used only if you can't get an MRI.

If you can get an MRI, do not use bone scan. A nuclear bone scan is a very sensitive test: It can "light up" with skin infection overlying the bone infection. Thus, a positive test is not helpful, especially if there might be cellulitis nearby or cancer in the bone. A negative test, on the other hand, is very helpful.

## Treatment

Try never to treat osteomyelitis empirically. Six weeks is a long time to wait to find you are wrong. Instead:

- Try to wait for a bone biopsy to be done before starting treatment.
- Give vancomycin or Zosyn while awaiting for results of biopsy.
- Gram-negative bacilli can be treated with oral ciprofloxacin if the organism is sensitive.
- IV antibiotics do not need to be given in the hospital itself; ertapenem or ceftriaxone can be given via IV once a day at home.
- X-ray, CT, and MRI cannot be used to follow the response to therapy.

# Acute Back Pain

The most urgent issue for acute back pain is to exclude serious pathology.

<table>
<tr><th>Cord Compression</th><th>Epidural Abscess</th><th>Cauda Equina</th><th>Disk Herniation</th></tr>
<tr><td>History of cancer</td><td>Fever, high ESR</td><td>Bowel and bladder incontinence, erectile dysfunction</td><td>Pain/numbness of medial calf or foot</td></tr>
<tr><td colspan="2">Vertebral tenderness, sensory level, hyperreflexia</td><td>Bilateral leg weakness, saddle area anesthesia</td><td>Loss of knee and ankle reflexes, positive straight leg raise</td></tr>
<tr><td>MRI<br>Steroid<br>Surgical decompression</td><td>Empirical antibiotics<br>Some surgery</td><td>Steroids</td><td>NSAIDs<br>Stretching and exercise</td></tr>
</table>

## Cord Compression

Look for back pain with:

- Hyperreflexia
- Vertebral tenderness
- Weakness
- Upgoing toes (extensor plantar reflex)
- Sensory "level": decrease in sensation below the point of compression

### Management of Cord Compression

When these conditions are present, this is a super emergency. To avert paralysis, you must:

1. Give 10 mg IV bolus of dexamethasone to reduce pressure/swelling on the spinal cord.
2. Get an MRI of the spine immediately.
3. Get an emergency neurology evaluation.
4. Evaluate for decompressive surgery.

> **Round Saver**
>
> Steroids fast is more important than waiting for the MRI.

## Benign Low Back Pain

"Benign" does not mean it is not serious or not painful. It means the patient will not be paralyzed and is not developing a permanent neurological deficit. Low back pain can be considered "benign" if:

- No focal neurological deficits
- No hyperreflexia
- No spine tenderness

An abnormal "straight leg raise" test on physical examination is not a "focal neurological deficit." An abnormal straight leg raise is simply a radiculopathy or peripheral neuropathy of the nerve root.

### Management of Benign Low Back Pain

1. NSAIDs (e.g., ibuprofen)
2. Stretching, yoga, chiropractic, acupuncture
3. Cyclobenzaprine, a muscle relaxant that can cause sleepiness

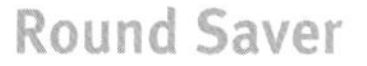


> Bed rest or an MRI is wrong for benign low back pain.

# Rheumatoid Arthritis (RA)

RA presents as:

- Multiple joints, small more often than large
- Symptoms lasting >6 weeks
- Morning stiffness >1 hour
- Elevated ESR or CRP
- Rheumatoid factor (RF) or anti-cyclic citrullinated peptide (anti-CCP)

Although nodules in skin can be present, they are not required to establish a diagnosis.

## Issues Specific to Inpatient Management

- C1/C2 cervical spine instability affects intubation: be careful about intubation
- Immunosuppressive medications cause infections
- RA can be cause of pericarditis
- RA can be the reason your patient got septic arthritis

**Round Saver**

You can break their neck! Be careful. This is real.

## Diagnostic Testing

- Normocytic anemia is extremely common
- RF is present in only 70% of patients and is not specific to RA
- Anti-CCP is extremely specific to RA
- X-rays do NOT have to be abnormal to have RA!

## Treatment

1. NSAIDs
2. Steroids briefly for acute exacerbations
3. Start disease-modifying anti-rheumatic drugs (DMARDs) early in the course of therapy

### Mechanism and Adverse Effects of DMARDs

| Medication | Mechanism | Adverse Effect |
|---|---|---|
| Methotrexate | Folate antagonist | Lung and liver fibrosis |
| Rituximab | Anti-CD20 | Infection |
| Etanercept, adalimumab | Anti-TNF | Reactivation of TB infection |
| Anakinra | IL-1 inhibitor Neutrophil activation | Infection |
| Abatacept | Stops T-cells | Infection |

# Systemic Lupus Erythematosus (SLE)

You need 4 of 11 criteria to establish a diagnosis of SLE; however, only a few of these issues lead to hospitalization.

- **Skin:**
  - Malar rash
  - Oral and vaginal ulcers
  - Discoid skin lesions
  - Photosensitivity
- **CNS:** Confusion/disorientation/stroke in young people
- **Heme:** Anemia, thrombocytopenia, neutropenia, or any combination

**Round Saver**

Anemia of chronic disease is more common than hemolysis in SLE.

- **Renal:** From mild proteinuria to hematuria to end-stage renal disease
- **Serositis:** Pleuritis or pericarditis
- **Joint:** Pain, but the x-ray and aspiration of the joint will be normal

## Issues Specific to Inpatient Management

Patients with SLE can be admitted for:

- Fever and chest pain from pericarditis
- Renal insufficiency
- Confusion, stroke, or encephalitis in a young person
- Clotting/thrombophilia from antiphospholipid syndrome

## Diagnostic Testing

- ANA: 95–99% sensitive
- Anti-double stranded DNA (dsDNA) 60% sensitive but nearly 100% specific
- Anti-Sm: specific, but we do not know what to do when it is positive
- Anti-Ro: neonatal SLE and likelihood of developing heart block

## Treatment

1. Glucocorticoids (e.g., prednisone or methylprednisolone) for acute flare of SLE
2. Hydroxychloroquine to prevent progression
3. Belimumab prevents progression by suppressing lymphocytes
4. Lupus nephritis: steroid and either cyclophosphamide or mycophenolate

**Round Saver**

Belimumab is the first new lupus drug in 50 years!

## Antiphospholipid (APL) Syndrome

There are two types of APL syndromes:

- Lupus anticoagulant
- Anti-cardiolipin antibody

Both present with abnormal clotting leading to:

- Pulmonary emboli (PE)
- Stroke, which can be in a young person
- Spontaneous abortion: 2 first-trimester or 1 second-trimester
- Infarction of peripheral arteries leading to loss of digits

### Diagnostic Testing

- Elevated aPTT with a normal INR and normal prothrombin time (PT)
- Mixing study: aPTT will not correct (come to normal) with APL syndrome
- Russell viper venom test: most specific test for lupus anticoagulant

### Treatment

Use heparin and warfarin as you would for any other clotting disorder. The goal of INR is 2–3 as it is in any clotting disorder. The only difference is that lifelong anticoagulation after a single clot is more likely to be used than in other clotting disorders.

**Round Saver**

APL syndrome has the highest likelihood of recurrence of any thrombophilia.

# Gout

Gout is frequently admitted with an acute flare resulting in:

- Extremely severe, sudden pain in the foot, toe, or knee
- Erythema
- Easily confused with septic arthritis or cellulitis

**Things You Will Be Asked on Rounds**

- Binge drinking? (beer is the worst)
- Red meat eaten?
- Thiazide diuretics? (increase uric acid level)
- Recent chemotherapy?

## Diagnostic Testing

Aspirate the joint for:

- Negatively birefringent crystals on polarizing microscope
- Synovial fluid: 10,000–20,000, predominantly neutrophils

## Treatment

Pain management is critical! For **acute therapy**, NSAIDs of any kind are the best initial therapy (e.g., ibuprofen, naproxen, sulindac). If there is renal insufficiency (thus contraindicating NSAIDs), use glucocorticoids.

- Intra-articular injection for single joint
- IV for multiple joints

**Round Saver**

Do **not** use allopurinol during an acute flare of gout!

Colchicine is used to prevent attacks. It was used as initial therapy for acute gout flare until only recently—forgive your attending if he is a little stuck in the past. Colchicine is still used if neither NSAIDs nor steroids can be used.

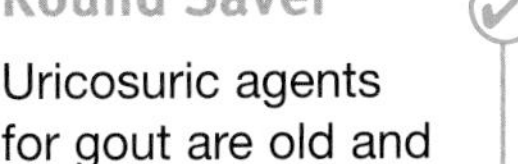


Uricosuric agents for gout are old and much less effective.

For **preventive therapy**, use allopurinol or febuxostat to decrease uric acid levels, and colchicine to prevent attacks.

- Rasburicase or pegloticase dissolves uric acid with few adverse effects
- Losartan is the best BP drug in gout. Losartan (an ARB) lowers uric acid levels.
- Probenecid and sulfinpyrazone are old, markedly less effective therapies to increase urine excretion of uric acid

## Pseudogout (Calcium Pyrophosphate Deposition Disease)

Pseudogout presents in much the same way as septic arthritis or gout as a joint that is hot, red, warm, swollen, and immobile. The difference is that pseudogout:

- Involves large joints such as the knee
- Is associated with hemochromatosis and hyperparathyroidism
- Has positively birefringent rhomboid shaped crystals
- Does not have an association with hyperuricemia
- Is not treated with allopurinol, febuxostat, or rasburicase

### Management

1. The first test is a joint aspiration
2. Most accurate test is arthrocentesis to find crystals
3. NSAIDs are the initial therapy
4. Intra-articular steroids (triamcinolone)
5. Colchicine for both acute therapy and prophylaxis in those with frequent attacks

## VASCULITIS

Vasculitis is an idiopathic inflammation of blood vessels. All forms can present with:

- Fever and weight loss
- Joint pain
- Skin lesions (e.g., petechiae or purpura)
- High ESR or CRP

Chronic versions have a normocytic anemia, leukocytosis, and thrombocytosis. Further manifestations depend on the specific type of vasculitis.

Vasculitis is most accurately diagnosed by biopsy. It is treated with glucocorticoids (e.g., prednisone) and, possibly, with cyclophosphamide subsequently.

### Wegener's Granulomatosis

Wegener's granulomatosis is a systemic vasculitis that presents with:

- Upper respiratory involvement (otitis media, sinusitis)
- Lung disease (non-resolving lung lesions)
- Renal: glomerulonephritis (hematuria, proteinuria)
- Skin: petechiae, purpura
- Joint pain

### Key to Diagnosis

Wegener's granulomatosis predominantly involves the respiratory system and the kidney. The patient will look like someone with pneumonia—there is fever, cough, sputum, hemoptysis, and an abnormal chest x-ray. But there is no improvement or resolution with antibiotics.

### Diagnostic Testing

1. Chest x-ray: nodules, adenopathy, cavities
2. Urinalysis: proteinuria, hematuria, and red cell casts
3. C-ANCA
4. Biopsy of the lung or kidney is the most accurate test

### Treatment

Glucocorticoids and cyclophosphamide have been the standard of care for many years.

## Churg-Strauss Syndrome

Look for the signs of vasculitis (weight loss, skin lesions, peripheral neuropathy, joint and muscle pain) in association with:

- Asthma not responsive to inhaled bronchodilators (95%)
- Eosinophilia
- Renal manifestations (30%)
- Mononeuritis multiplex (70%)
- Cardiac (50–70%)

**Round Saver** 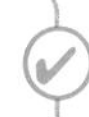

Churg-Strauss = vasculitis with asthma + eosinophils

### Diagnostic Testing

All types of vasculitis give a high ESR, CRP, and normocytic anemia. Beside eosinophils, the most characteristic finding of Churg-Strauss syndrome is a P-ANCA also known as anti-myeloperoxidase (anti-MPO).

The single most accurate test is biopsy of lung or kidney.

### Treatment

1. Glucocorticoids (prednisone)
2. Cyclophosphamide
3. Replace cyclophosphamide with azathioprine, mycophenolate, or methotrexate

## Microscopic Polyangiitis (MPA)

- Lung and renal manifestations, fever, weight loss, peripheral neuropathy, joint and muscle pain
- **No granulomas** (*UNLIKE* Wegener's)
- **No eosinophils or asthma** (*UNLIKE* Churg-Strauss)
- Anemia, high ESR, and CRP (ANCA-positive)
- Biopsy most accurate test
- Steroids and cyclophosphamide

## Polyarteritis Nodosa (PAN)

PAN spares the lung and is associated with hepatitis B and C. Angiography or the GI and renal vessels can eliminate the need for renal biopsy.

PAN has the same manifestations of vasculitis as MPA, Churg-Strauss, and Wegener's such as fever, weight loss, joint and muscle pain, renal, skin, and GI abnormalities. The ESR and CRP are up, but the hematocrit is down. The most accurate test is a biopsy.

Treatment is steroids. If steroids do not work, add cyclophosphamide.

## Takayasu's Arteritis

Look for fever, fatigue, weight loss, joint and muscle pain plus:

- Asian women <40 years old
- Decreased pulses of arms and legs

Testing is angiography (MRA). Biopsy is not routinely done, as these are large arteries. Treat with steroids; use methotrexate or azathioprine for steroid-resistant cases.

## Polymyalgia Rheumatica (PMR)

### Presentation

Presents in patients > age 50 (average 70) with:

- Pain in proximal muscles without tenderness on examination
- Hips, shoulders, neck "stiffness" and "aching" worse in the morning
- Symptoms making it difficult to dress or get up from bed
- Decreased range of motion
- Pain and stiffness, NOT decreased motor strength

> **Round Saver**
>
> PMR is distinctly **non**-tender!

## Testing and Treatment

- Elevated ESR and C-reactive protein (CRP)
- Normocytic anemia
- Normal ANA, CPK, aldolase, and myoglobin
- Prednisone at low dose (20 mg/day) gives an extremely brisk and satisfying improvement over hours

**Round Saver**

PMR is pain and stiffness without destruction.

# Giant Cell (Temporal) Arteritis (GCA)

The presence of 3 of the following 5 criteria have >90% sensitivity and specificity for GCA:

- >50 years old
- Headache of new onset
- Jaw claudication (pain in jaw on chewing)
- Visual symptoms (e.g., amaurosis fugax, retinal artery occlusion, diplopia)
- Tenderness over temporal artery
- ESR >50 mm/hour or increased CRP
- Biopsy of temporal artery

**Round Saver**

Don't wait for biopsy results to start steroids.

**Round Saver**

ESR and CRP are essentially interchangeable

## Henoch-Schönlein Purpura (HSP)

HSP is IgA deposited in vessels throughout the body, but the symptoms are localized to:

- **GI:** pain, nausea, vomiting, diarrhea, bleeding, intussusception
- **Joint:** arthralgia
- **Skin:** purpuric lesions on buttocks and legs; raised, nonblanching
- **Renal:** proteinuria, hematuria, RBC casts; rare progression to nephritic

### Testing and Treatment

Although biopsy is the most accurate test, this is rarely needed. IgA levels are often done, but are normal in 50%. Skin biopsy is easier than kidney biopsy.

HSP is a "controversial" disease. Acknowledge this by saying "My understanding is that biopsy and steroids are controversial. What do you feel is best?"

> **Round Saver**
>
> It is always better to say "This is what I think is right, do you agree or disagree?" rather than "Tell me what to do."

"Severe HSP" =

- Inability to take fluids
- Rising BUN and creatinine
- Severe abdominal pain not responsive to NSAIDs

Treatment:

1. NSAIDs (e.g., Naprosyn) are the mainstay of therapy.
2. Prednisone if there is severe disease that is progressing. Using steroids for progressing disease is very different from using them to prevent renal failure with normal kidneys.

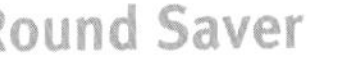


> No blood test confirms HSP. No treatments clearly **prevent** progression to renal failure.

## Cryoglobulinemia

- Circulating antibodies
- Associated with chronic hepatitis C
- **Renal:** glomerulonephritis (30–60%)
- **Joint:** arthralgia
- **Skin:** purpura

**Round Saver** 

Cryoglobulins rarely give GI symptoms

### Testing

- Cryoglobulin level
- Rheumatoid factor positive in nearly 100%
- Complement levels low

**Round Saver** 

Cold agglutinins: hemolysis

Cryoglobulins: renal, joint, skin

### Treatment

- Secondary cryoglobulinemia: treat underlying cause (e.g., hepatitis C)
- "Essential mixed" cryoglobulinemia: steroids and sometimes plasmapheresis work

## Behcet's Syndrome

Behcet's disease is an idiopathic constellation of mucocutaneous lesions with severe ocular disease in Middle Eastern men. There is no blood or radiologic testing.

- Oral ulcers
- Genital lesions
- Ocular disease (uveitis) that can lead to blindness
- Skin hypersensitivity: pathergy
- Arthritis
- Treat with colchicine; use steroids for those not responding.

# SERONEGATIVE SPONDYLOARTHROPATHIES

These are diseases with joint pain and often joint deformity, but a negative rheumatoid factor. There is no specific blood test for any of them. All are treated with NSAIDs; severe forms get methotrexate (psoriatic) or anti-TNF drugs (ankylosing spondylitis and reactive arthritis).

## Ankylosing Spondylitis

Ankylosing spondylitis (AS) is a disease of young men starting in their 20s and 30s. The diagnosis is often delayed for 1–2 years after the onset of back pain because at first there are no physical findings and the x-ray can be normal. There is also no blood test.

When a 25-year-old man comes to the office saying "I have back pain," few practitioners immediately make the leap: "You must have a chronic incurable progressive source of permanent disability and pain—let's MRI your sacroiliac joint." Hence the delay.

Look for back pain in a young man with:

- Radiation to the buttocks and the legs
- Hip pain
- Improvement with exercise and stretching
- Enthesitis: inflammation of attachment points of tendons
- Progressive immobility
- Schober test: fixed lumbar vertebrae that do not expand when bending over

**Advanced disease** presents with:

- Restrictive lung disease
- Eye findings (uveitis) in 30–40%
- Aortic valve disease (2–3%)

### Diagnostic Testing

1. X-ray of sacroiliac (SI) joint
2. MRI of SI joints is more sensitive
3. HLA-B27 testing is not useful since 8% of the general population is positive

### Treatment

1. NSAIDs
2. Anti-TNF drugs (infliximab, etanercept, adalimumab)

**Round Saver** 

Steroids should NOT be used in AS.

## Psoriatic Arthritis

A small fraction of those with psoriasis (<10%) will develop arthritis. The extent of psoriatic skin involvement is not correlated to the likelihood of developing arthritis. It can happen with even a tiny amount of skin disease. Presentation:

- Distal interphalangeal oligoarthritis
- Nail pitting
- Enthesitis (inflammation of tendinous insertion points)
- High ESR/CRP with all other tests normal
- "Pencil-in-cup" deformity on x-ray

### Treatment

1. NSAIDs first
2. Methotrexate
3. If methotrexate does not control disease use anti-TNF medications, sulfasalazine or hydroxychloroquine

## Reactive Arthritis (Reiter Syndrome)

Joint pain and deformity can occur as a "reaction" to:

- Chlamydial infection
- Inflammatory bowel disease
- Gastrointestinal infection

This is an oligoarthritis, often of the knees. It is associated with:

- Eye lesions (conjunctivitis, uveitis)
- Genital lesion (balanitis)

### Treatment

Use NSAIDs and treat the underlying associated disease if there is one. Use sulfasalazine if the disorder does not resolve with NSAIDs and treating the underlying cause.

## Adult Still's Disease (Juvenile Rheumatoid Arthritis)

Still's disease is a febrile illness with joint pain, rash, big spleen, and pericarditis. Lab tests show a leukocytosis with >10,000–15,000 neutrophils, normocytic anemia, and leukocytosis. Reactive thrombocytosis is common.

| | |
|---|---|
| S | ***S***plenomegaly |
| T | ***T***emperature, ***T***hrombocytosis |
| I | ***I***ll patient |
| L | ***L***ymph nodes |
| L | ***L***eukocytosis, ***L***iver enzymes |
| S | ***S***almon rash |

There is no single diagnostic test, although a markedly elevated ferritin level occurs in 75%. Treat with aspirin or NSAIDs. Those not responding get steroids. Occasional patients need an anti-TNF drug.

## Spinal Stenosis

This is narrowing of the spinal canal with a hypertrophied ligamentum flavum. Look for:

- Age >60 with back pain radiating down buttocks and thighs
- Worse walking down hill or stairs or anything leaning back
- Better leaning forward (cycling)
- Mimics vascular disease! Vascular disease pain is with exertion in any direction
- Ankle/brachial index (ABI) normal in spinal stenosis
- MUST have MRI

### Treatment

1. Lose weight, exercise, stretch, cycle, swim
2. NSAIDs and pain meds
3. Epidural steroid shots
4. Surgical decompression (laminectomy) if these other measures do not work

## Osteoarthritis

Look for older patients with multiple joint involvement. Osteoarthritis is typically a pain of overuse, so it will worsen during the day. Rheumatoid arthritis gets better with use. Look for pain in:

- Knees
- Hips
- Hands, particularly worsened with use

## Diagnostic Testing

All blood tests are normal. If the ESR or CRP is abnormal, look for another diagnosis. The problem with ANA is that 5% of general population has an ANA positive, so a positive ANA test can be confusing.

> **Round Saver**
>
> Don't submit ANA test results unless features of SLE other than joint pain are present.

X-rays show joint narrowing because articular cartilage is mostly water. When watery cartilage is gone, the bones look close together or appear to be touching. Osteophyte presence by itself means little. Pain with no osteophytes can still be OA. Osteophytes without pain are meaningless.

## Treatment

1. Acetaminophen first. NSAIDs work, but this is a chronic disease; 20% of those using continuous NSAIDs for a year will have an ulcer. There is no point in burning a hole in someone's guts with an NSAID for no extra efficacy at first.
2. Capsaicin cream
3. Weight loss and exercise. The stronger your muscles, the less work your joint must do. The lighter you are, the less work the joints must do.
4. Intra-articular steroids (triamcinolone) or hyaluronic acid: patients will love it, but it needs an injection and it only lasts a few weeks. If the patient needs these, they are heading toward joint replacement.

## Fibromyalgia

Pain disorder without any objective laboratory findings. Patients have:

- Muscle and joint pain
- Multiple tender "trigger points." Some are in hard to understand areas like the medial fat pad of the knee.
- By definition all lab tests and radiology are normal.
- Treat with duloxetine, pregabalin, gabapentin, tricyclic antidepressants (e.g., amitriptyline or milnacipran).
- Look for depression to treat.
- Exercise programs really help.

## Carpal Tunnel Syndrome

The defining feature is hand pain of the thumb, index, and middle finger that gets worse with repetitive exercise. The pain is worse at night.

- Tinel's: pain with tapping on the median nerve
- Phalen's: pain with extreme flexion of the wrists

Wasting of thumb muscles occur with severe disease.

Carpal tunnel is associated with swelling of the nerve or soft tissue of the wrist such as occurs with:

- Pregnancy
- Diabetes, hypothyroidism, or acromegaly
- Amyloidosis
- Rheumatoid arthritis

### Testing

Specific testing is usually not necessary. The most accurate test is nerve conduction velocity or electromyography.

### Treatment

1. Wrist splints and getting the right equipment when using computer keyboards
2. Physical therapy, yoga
3. Steroid injections
4. Surgical decompression by cutting the flexor retinaculum

## Dupuytren Contracture

- Flexion contracture of the 4th and 5th fingers in the flexor tendons of the hand.
- Immobility and nodules of the tendons
- No tests available
- Early disease: inject collagenase
- Advancing disease: inject triamcinolone (steroid) or lidocaine
- Surgery for release if progression cannot be stopped

## Rotator Cuff Injury

- Pain in the lateral shoulder that is worse at night
- Pain worsened with work that lifts the arm over the head
- Ask the patient to lift arm overhead from the side with you pressing against it. Rotator cuff injury causes lots of pain when it goes overhead
- MRI is the test. X-ray and ultrasound have almost no benefit.
- Acute, full tears need immediate surgery
- Chronic, partial tears get physical therapy and steroid injections

# Plantar Fasciitis

- Severe pain in bottom of foot near heel
- Worst in morning
- Improves with a few steps
- X-rays useless; bone spurs common in general population
- Treat with stretching, ice, and NSAIDs
- Steroid injection if not improving
- Surgical release of fascia rarely needed

# Scleroderma (Systemic Sclerosis)

## Limited Disease (CREST Syndrome)

**C**alcinosis, **R**aynaud's, **E**sophageal dysmotility, **S**clerodactyly, and **T**elangiectasia seems self-explanatory as a disease with such an excellent acronym. Patients present with skin changes and:

- GERD symptoms of heartburn
- Ulcerations of fingers
- Primary pulmonary hypertension leading to dyspnea

CREST is diagnosed by the presence of the syndrome and anti-centromere antibodies.

### Treatment of CREST

- Skin lesions: nothing clearly delays progression
- Raynaud's: calcium channel blockers
- GERD: proton-pump inhibitors
- Pulmonary hypertension:
  - Bosentan, ambrisentan: endothelin antagonists
  - Sildenafil
  - Prostacyclin analogues: epoprostenol, treprostinil, iloprost

## Diffuse (Systemic) Scleroderma

Diffuse disease has all the findings of CREST as well as:

- Renal disease: treat hypertensive crisis with ACE inhibitors
- Cardiomyopathy
- Lung fibrosis (not just the pulmonary artery): treat with cyclophosphamide
- SCL-70 antibodies are present in 30%

# Polymyositis and Dermatomyositis

- Proximal muscle weakness: cannot rise from seated position without using hands
- Skin lesions:
    - Gottron's papules: back of hands
    - Heliotrope rash: around the eyes
- Muscle destruction
- Elevated CPK and elevated aldolase level
- Elevated ESR and CRP
- Anti-Jo antibody: predicts lung involvement
- Muscle biopsy: most accurate test
- **Must exclude cancer!!!!**
- Treat with steroids
- Methotrexate, azathioprine and IVIG if not responsive to steroids

**Round Saver**

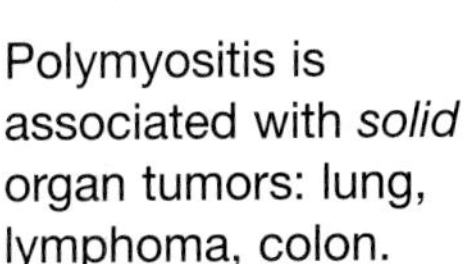

Polymyositis is associated with *solid* organ tumors: lung, lymphoma, colon.

**Round Saver**

Anti-Jo antibodies predict lung involvement.

# Sjögren's Syndrome

Sjögren's is quite common in middle-aged women. Although the most common symptom is joint pain, this is not specific enough to lead to a diagnosis. For a diagnosis of Sjögren's, look for:

- Dry eyes, mouth, and vagina:
  - "Do you fell sand in your eyes?"
  - "Do you have to wake up at night to drink water?"
- Recurrent dental caries (cavities) from the mouth dryness
- Recurrent sinus disease
- Lymphoma develops

**Round Saver**

Lymphoma is the most dangerous long-term complication of Sjögren.

## Diagnostic Testing

- ANA: found in >90% but nonspecific; negative ANA goes strongly against Sjögren's syndrome
- SSA (Ro)/SSB (La): 40–50% but fairly specific for the disease
- Schirmer's test: inability to wet filter paper placed into the eye
- Rose Bengal: abnormal staining of conjunctivae from dryness
- Salivary gland scintigraphy, sialography (the duct), or MRI
- Salivary gland biopsy: single most accurate test

**Round Saver** 

Yes, there really is a test called "tear breakup time."

## Treatment

1. Artificial tears and saliva, sour sugar-free candy
2. Pilocarpine and cevimeline increase salivary secretions
3. Hydroxychloroquine for arthralgias
4. Steroids do not work

# Afterword

"Thank you for saving my life. If it wasn't for all of you, I would be dead right now."

It's Friday afternoon and rounds are done. The labs are checked, the notes are written. All the right medications have been ordered, and all the patients are comfortable.

The medicine was done right.

A man from one of the best hotels in Manhattan has had his catheterization, and the pain of an acute myocardial infarction is gone.

Too soon, the team flows out of the patient's room. "Let's stop for a second," I say. "Did you all *really* hear what that man said? 'Thank you for saving my life'?"

"Wow," they say. It sinks in. Everything we do *matters.*

Our lives are not wasted; we have more meaning. *We have mastered the Wards.*

And we all leave the hospital feeling . . . *happy.*

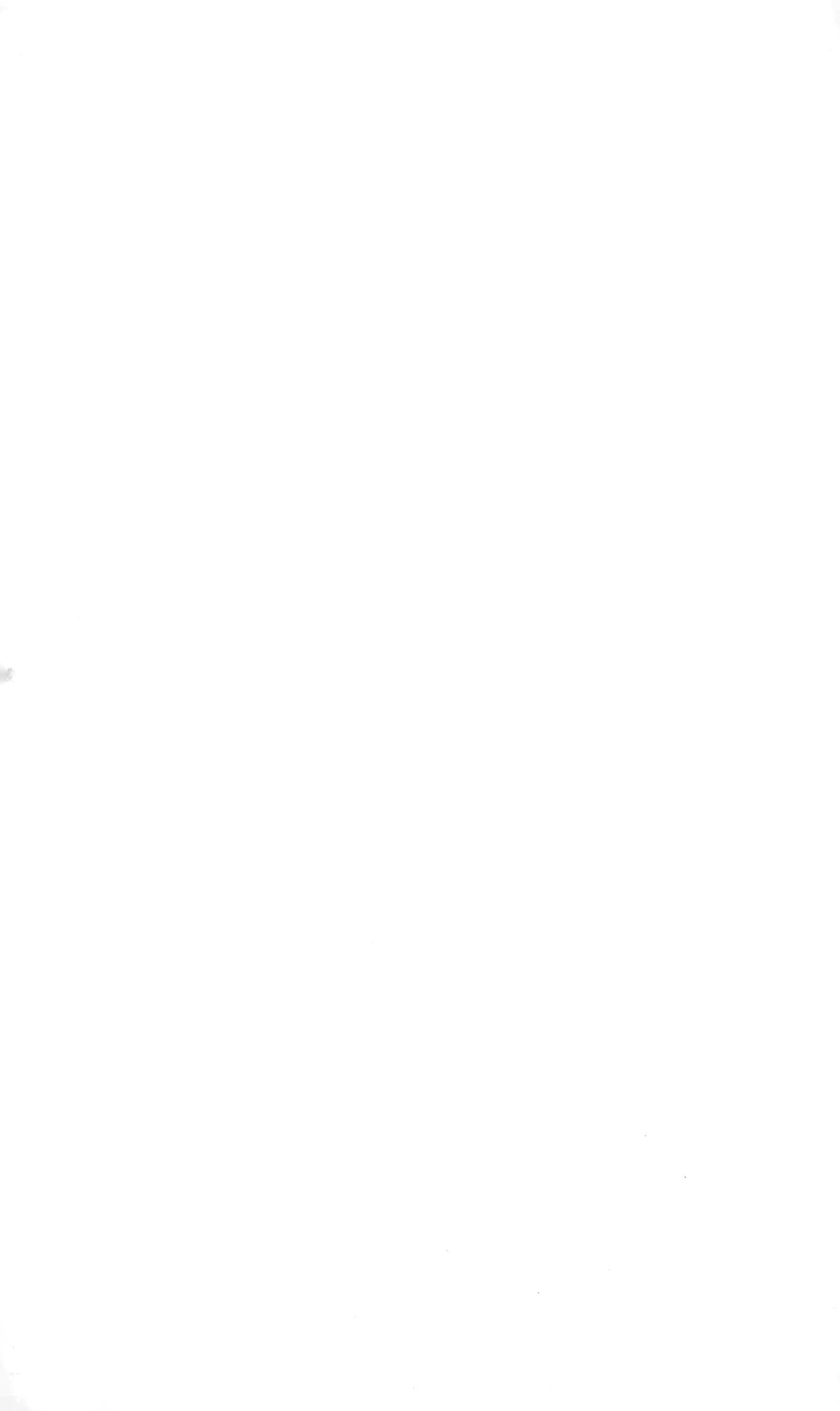

# About the Author

**Conrad Fischer, MD,** is director of educational development for the Department of Medicine at Jamaica Hospital Medical Center in New York City. Jamaica Hospital is a robust window on the world of medicine. Dr. Fischer is also chairman of medicine for Kaplan Medical, teaching USMLE Steps 1, 2, and 3; Internal Medicine Board Review and Attending Recertification; and USMLE Step 1 Physiology. Dr. Fischer is associate professor of physiology, pharmacology, and medicine at Touro College of Osteopathic Medicine in New York City.